Fundamentals
of
Cardiac
Surgery

Fundamentals
of
Cardiac
Surgery

Charles Marks

Professor of Surgery Emeritus
Louisiana State University Medical School
Louisiana, USA

Consultant Cardiothoracic Surgeon
Parirenyatwa Hospital, Ministry of Health, Harare, Zimbabwe

Formerly Senior Attending Surgeon
Charity Hospital, Veterans Administration Hospital,
Hotel Dieu and Touro Infirmary, New Orleans, Louisiana, USA

Formerly Hunterian Professor
Royal College of Surgeons of England

Peter H. Marks

Chief Cardiothoracic Surgeon
The Rockford Clinic, Rockford, Illinois, USA

Clinical Instructor
University of Illinois Medical School, Rockford, Illinois, USA

CHAPMAN & HALL MEDICAL
London · Glasgow · New York · Tokyo · Melbourne · Madras

Published by Chapman & Hall, 2–6 Boundary Row, London SE1 8HN

Chapman & Hall, 2–6 Boundary Row, London SE1 8HN, UK

Blackie Academic & Professional, Wester Cleddens Road, Bishopbriggs, Glasgow G65 2NZ, UK

Chapman & Hall Inc., 29 West 35th Street, New York NY 10001, USA

Chapman & Hall Japan, Thomson Publishing Japan, Hirakawacho Nemoto Building, 6F, 1–7–11 Hirakawa-cho, Chiyoda-ku, Tokyo 102, Japan

Chapman & Hall Australia, Thomas Nelson Australia, 102 Dodds Street, South Melbourne, Victoria 3205, Australia

Chapman & Hall India, R. Seshadri, 32 Second Main Road, CIT East, Madras 600 035, India

First edition 1993

© 1993 Charles Marks and Peter H. Marks

Typeset by TextPertise (Private) Limited, Harare, Zimbabwe
Printed in Great Britain at the University Press, Cambridge.

ISBN 0 412 54310 9

A catalogue record for this book is available from the British Library

Library of Congress Cataloging-in-Publication data available

Contents

Foreword

Cardiac surgery is now an acceptable therapeutic procedure for many cardiac conditions both congenital and acquired.

Although this statement is not questioned in most western nations, thousands of treatable patients with cardiac disease die in Africa and other underdeveloped countries due to the total lack of facilities for the most simple forms of cardiac surgery.

This is now slowly but surely being remedied. The authors of *Fundamentals of Cardiac Surgery* have succeeded in producing an excellent textbook in anticipation of the need for training cardiac surgeons, nurses and other medical personnel to ensure well-trained staff to perform this much needed cardiac surgery at a high standard.

This textbook succeeds in its object to summarize the various aspects of cardiac surgery. Students and cardiac residents will find the text easy to read and to understand. Although written in a summarized form the information is more than adequate. Nursing personnel and pump technicians will also benefit from studying this textbook.

For the cardiac surgeon and cardiologist, *Fundamentals of Cardiac Surgery* offers easy reference and excellent information before operations or refreshes some forgotten details.

After nearly 30 years as a cardiac surgeon I not only enjoyed reading every page but became excited by all the developments over the past few decades in cardiac surgery and the challenges of the future.

Fundamentals of Cardiac Surgery is an excellent textbook and highly recommended to be read and studied by those of us entrusted with the care of the cardiac conditions of our people.

Marius Barnard
Milpark Hospital
Johannesburg

Preface

The spectacular advances in the diagnosis and surgical treatment of complex congenital heart defects and acquired heart disease have spawned a vast bibliography and many encyclopaedic treatises on the various interrelated disciplines that are so necessary for effective cure or amelioration of the disorders that can afflict the heart.

This volume does not presume to be a definitive text in cardiac surgery. It is our aim to summarize the various aspects of the field with integration of the basic sciences and available clinical and operative information in a concise manner that will provide an overview of current practice.

It is directed to students, surgical residents and registrars and to the many diverse members of the open-heart units. Nursing personnel, pump technicians and cardiologists at all levels of training and attainment may find the information helpful in the course of their interface with cardiac surgeons.

Details of surgical operative procedures have been emphasized so that students and house staff can refresh their memories regarding the case at hand as they prepare to observe or assist at the respective operative procedures.

Acknowledgements

We are grateful to the many medical students, registrars and resident surgeons, in the United Kingdom, United States and Southern Africa, to whom we lectured over the past two decades on "Fundamentals of Cardiac Surgery". These lectures have served as the basis for this book.

We wish to express our appreciation to Mr C. T. Faranisi, FRCS, and Dr G. Hyde, MD, FACS, of the Department of Surgery, University of Zimbabwe, for their review of the manuscript. We are especially grateful to Sir Terence English, PRCS, Cambridge, England, Professor N. Oldham, MD, FACS, Duke University Medical Centre, USA, and Dr M. Barnard, Ch.M., FACS, Milpark Hospital, Johannesburg, for their gracious critiques and advice.

Although their recommendations have been implemented, any residual errors of omission or commission remain the fault of the authors.

We are deeply appreciative for the Foreword written by Dr Marius Barnard, whose contributions to cardiac surgery are universally appreciated.

We wish to thank Mrs J. Marks and the University of Zimbabwe art department for the illustrative details.

PART I
GENERAL CARDIOVASCULAR DISORDER

Chapter 1
Cardiovascular Collapse

Cardiac arrest is defined as cessation of an effective circulation due to:
a) Cardiac asystole
b) Ventricular fibrillation
c) Inadequate cardiac output due to:
   i) Bradycardia
   ii) Tachycardia
   iii) Poor myocardial contractility

Aetiology
1 Myocardial anoxia:
   a) Coronary artery occlusion
   b) Anoxia (airway obstruction; hypoventilation)
2 Reflex: vasovagal
3 Drugs, electrolyte disorder or acidosis:
   a) Overdose of digitalis, quinidine; procainamide
   b) Anaesthetic agents: chloroform, cyclopropane, halothane, cocaine
   c) Potassium (high or low levels), calcium (high levels)
   d) Acidosis: metabolic or respiratory
4 Diagnosis of cardiac arrest:
   a) Unconsciousness
   b) Apnoea
   c) Absent pulses
   d) Dilating pupil

Treatment
1 Provision for cardiopulmonary resuscitation:
   a) External cardiac massage
   b) Artificial ventilation
     i) Mouth to mouth respiration
     ii) Ambu bag
     iii) Endotracheal tube

2   Connect patient to ECG machine to determine whether cause is: asystole, arrhythmia or ventricular fibrillation.
3   Medical therapy: establish intravenous line:
   a) Sodium bicarbonate (80 mE per 15 minutes of arrest) counters the metabolic acidosis
   b) Adrenalin 10 ml of 1/10 000 solution and calcium chloride: 10 ml of 2% solution: improves heart tone
   c) Reduce myocardial irritability: lignocaine: 100 mg bolus; potassium chloride: 40 mE
   d) Vasopressors: dopamine, dobutamine.
4   Electrical defibrillation: restore normal rhythm by a shock of 200 J from a direct current defibrillator. It will abort an episode of ventricular fibrillation. Temporary pacemaker may be necessary.
5   Monitor patient:
   a) Vital signs: pulse, respiration, blood pressure
   b) Oscilloscope for cardiac rhythm
   c) Oxygen administration
   d) Nasogastric tube to prevent aspiration
   e) Urinary catheter
   f) Central venous pressure line
6   Treatment of complications:
   a) Cerebral damage: Dexamethasone
   b) Respiratory failure: mechanical ventilation; blood gases
   c) Renal failure: frusemide, ion-exchange resins; dialysis.

Heart failure

Heart failure can be defined as a condition in which ventricular output can only match venous return after substantial increase in filling pressure.

The failure may be left ventricular alone or right ventricular only. Congestive cardiac failure exists when biventricular failure occurs.

The pathophysiologic mechanisms causing heart failure are:
   a) Preload: volume overload necessitates high volume output
   b) Afterload: pressure overload increases ventricular work against an increased pressure.

c) Ventricular muscle dysfunction: cardiomegaly or myocardial ischaemia.

d) Arrhythmias: May lead to left ventricular failure.

Right ventricular failure

Preload: Volume overload; atrial septal defect; tricuspid incompetence.

Afterload: Pressure overload in pulmonary stenosis; pulmonary hypertension.

Myocardial dysfunction: Endomyocardial fibrosis; myocardial amyloidosis.

Treatment of acute ventricular failure

1 Sit patient up and administer 100% oxygen.
2 Diuretics to reduce preload: frusemide 80 mg i.v. stat.
3 Digitalize: positive inotropic action.
4 Arrhythmia control a) drugs b) cardioversion.
5 Opiates: intravenous morphine reduces left ventricular and diastolic pressure in addition to its sedative effect.
6 Aminophyllin: a bronchodilator that also has inotropic and choronotropic effects on the heart.
7 Vasodilators: reduction of afterload will improve cardiac stroke volume.
   a) Sodium nitroprusside (nipride) reduces pre and afterload
   b) Glyceryl trinitrate and other long-acting nitrates reduces preload
   c) Captopril: reduction of angiotension II and aldosterone reduces sodium and water as well as being vasodilatory
   d) Reduction of afterload: hydralazine, prazosin; Beta-blockers (propranolol); calcium channel blockers (verapamil).
8 Reduction of circulating blood volume:
   a) Venesection with removal of a pint of blood reduces preload rapidly
   b) Rotating tourniquets reduce venous return and thus preload
   c) Haemodialysis or ultrafiltration will reduce preload.
9 Support of the failing heart:
   a) Intra-aortic balloon pump

b) Extracorporeal circulatory support

c) Left ventricular assist device.

Further Reading

Braunwald, E., Ross, J. Jnr, Sonneblick, E. H. Mechanisms of contraction of the normal and failing heart. *New Eng. J. Med.* 277: 962, 1967.

Foley, W. T. *Advances in management of cardiac disease.* Vol 1. Chicago: Yearbook Medical Publishers, 1980.

Levine, H. D. *Cardiac emergencies and related disorders. Their mechanisms, recognition and management.* New York: Appleton-Century-Crofts Inc., 1960.

Lown, B. Cardiovascular collapse and sudden death. In: Braunwald, E. (ed.). *Heart disease.* Philadelphia: W. B. Saunders, 1984.

McIntyre, K. M., Parker, M. R. Standards and guidelines for cardiopulmonary resuscitation (CPR) and emergency cardiac care (ECC). *JAMA* 244: 453, 1980.

Smith, T. W., Braunwald, E. The management of heart failure. In: Braunwald, E. (ed.) *Heart disease.* Philadelphia: W. B. Saunders. 503, 1984.

Chapter 2
Intra-aortic Balloon Pump

Insertion of this supportive device is indicated in the treatment of circulatory failure due to left ventricular myocardial ischaemia, as it reduces myocardial oxygen consumption. It may also be used in non-ischaemic causes of circulatory failure.

The device is appropriate in cases of pre-infarction angina with poor left ventricular function that may be improved after a subsequent aortocoronary bypass.

The use of the balloon pump may be life-saving in a patient with myocardial infarction who develops mitral insufficiency and in whom mitral valve reconstruction or replacement is subsequently feasible.

Circulatory failure due to a post-infarction interventricular septal rupture may, similarly, be supported by the intra-aortic balloon pump until repair of the acquired septal defect can be accomplished.

The procedure is also suitable for the postoperative cardiac surgery patient who may require the balloon pump to tide over temporary poor left ventricular function. Failure to wean the patient from cardiopulmonary bypass after open heart surgery may occasionally occur despite the use of inotropic agents (dobutamine or dobutrex) and vasodilators (nipride or nitroglycerine). Introduction of an intra-aortic balloon pump provides a safe method of increasing cardiac output by as much as 0.5 l per minute per square metre and may permit separation from bypass with support of cardiac function.

Technique
The device may consist of a 40 ml balloon on a 14F catheter or a 20 ml balloon on a 12F catheter.

The balloon sheath is inserted percutaneously over a flexible guidewire in the femoral artery after the entrance site has been dilated to a size 12 diameter.

The furled balloon is inserted through the sheath and is carefully advanced to the distal aortic arch below the left subclavian artery origin.

The balloon is designed to inflate during diastole and to deflate during systole. The balloon mechanism is triggered electronically by the patient's electrocardiogram with the timing sequence based on the R wave. With balloon deflation there is reduction in the heart's afterload. With balloon inflation in diastole there is an increase in diastolic pressure and in coronary blood flow.

Compromise of lower limb circulation may occur during the procedure and its regular monitoring is essential.

When judged appropriate the balloon is removed by deflating and withdrawing it from the groin. Manual pressure is applied to the arterial site for 20 minutes, followed by sandbag pressure for 6 hours.

The patient remains in bed for 24 hours with frequent review of the limb for reactionary haemorrhage that might require suture or for circulatory inadequacy that may require exploration, thrombectomy and Fogarty catheter clearance of the artery.

If the atherosclerotic occlusion of both femoral arteries precludes the percutaneous procedure, the balloon may be inserted directly into the aortic arch and properly positioned.

Ventricular assist device

The inability to separate a patient from cardiopulmonary bypass with drugs or an intra-aortic balloon pump may require a left atrial to aortic assist system. After 5 to 7 days of such support, cardiac function may be adequately restored. Closure of a patent foramen ovale is imperative to prevent a right to left shunt before inserting the device.

The heart is elevated and retracted to the right. Two purse-string sutures are inserted in the base of the left atrial appendage and the tipped cannula is inserted through an incision and secured. The cannula is filled with saline solution, clamped and brought through a subcostal tunnel. It is attached to the suction line of the pump oxygenator.

The dacron graft component of the composite arterial cannula is anastomosed to the side of the ascending aorta, filled with saline, clamped and brought through the subcostal tunnel.

The pump is attached and de-aired. When it has been activated, cardiopulmonary bypass is gradually stopped. The chest is then closed in the standard manner.

Right ventricular failure can be similarly supported by right atrium to pulmonary artery support.

Subsequent removal of the assist device will require re-sternotomy, discontinuance of pump action, with clamping and removal of atrial and aortic cannulae and the pump. After placement of chest tubes, closure of the sternotomy is accomplished.

Pacemaker insertion

Cardiac pacing is a very good mode of therapy for a variety of cardiac rhythm disorders.

The pacemaker is a device consisting of a pulse generator that has pacing and sensing capabilities. The generator and the cardiac electrodes or leads permit the delivery of a small electric current to atrium or ventricle in order to stimulate contraction.

Indications

1 Stokes–Adams attacks due to heart block
2 Slow ventricular rates refractory to medical therapy e.g. the sick sinus syndrome (tachycardia–bradycardia syndrome)
3 Complete heart block in myocardial ischaemia
4 Surgically induced complete heart block
5 Termination of tachyarrhythmia if anti-arrhythmic drugs have failed.

Temporary pacing

A temporary pacing electrode is introduced via the subclavian vein by the supra or infraclavicular route or via the internal jugular vein under local infiltration anaesthesia.

It is guided towards the heart where it tends to coil in the right atrium. The electrode is rotated clockwise and withdrawn slightly so that, under fluoroscopic control, it will be seen to be propelled through the tricuspid valve into the right ventricle, where it is positioned amongst the trabeculae.

The two leads are then attached to the generator and set at:
a) 70 beats per minute
b) 3 volts
c) On demand: the impulse is generated only if there is no inherent myocardial activity.

The threshold is measured so that the pacing complex is attained with the lowest possible voltage, usually less than 1 V.

The pacing wire is secured to the skin by suture, to prevent its accidental dislodgement.

Permanent pacing

Under 1% lidocaine local anaesthesia the cephalic vein is dissected out in the deltopectoral groove and the pacing wire passed and secured in the right ventricle.

A subcutaneous pouch is then created in the subpectoral region, so that there is no interference with shoulder movement. The generator is placed within this pouch. The subcutaneous tissues and the skin are then serially sutured. A low threshold is then established.

Modern generators are powered by lithium batteries that should last 7 years.

Epicardial leads may be placed temporarily on the atrium and ventricle after completion of open heart operative procedures, in anticipation of possible serious, though transitory, arrhythmias.

Rarely, permanent epicardial lead placement may be necessary via a left anterior thoracotomy. Two leads are usually placed, in case one becomes detached.

Dual-chamber pacing

One lead is introduced into the right atrial appendage and one into the right ventricle.

Types of pacing
1 *Fixed-rate asynchronous pacing:* These units stimulate the ventricles at a constant rhythm regardless of underlying cardiac rhythm or physiological requirements. Such units are not usually used for permanent pacing as pacer rhythms may conflict with changing conducted rhythms. Although this competition is generally harmless, it may rarely induce ventricular arrhythmias such as ventricular tachycardia or even ventricular fibrillation.
2 *Standby or demand pacing:* These fixed-rate units detect the ventricular R wave and do not stimulate until a preset time interval has elapsed. Pacing does not occur until the spontaneous

ventricular rate falls below the preset minimum interval. During periods of normal sinus rhythm an implanted demand pacemaker is inhibited.
3 *Synchronous (variable-rate) pacing:* These units are designed to stimulate the ventricles in response to an atrial signal received through a separate sensing circuit. It responds to normal variations of sinus rhythm. The unit is appropriate for younger patients with heart block whose intact myocardium permits a maximal physiological response to activity.

Although pacing originally depended on bipolar lead stimulation with a positive anode and a negative cathode both in the heart, a unipolar system with the cathode in the heart and the anode in the subcutaneous tissue near the generator has proven to be preferable.

Cardioversion

An external direct current countershock is an effective method for terminating many cardiac arrhythmias that are life-threatening, e.g. ventricular tachycardia, or cause a low cardiac output syndrome refractory to medical therapy.

Synchronous or asynchronous shock: to avoid a shock during the T wave of the cardiac cycle, a synchronized shock is predetermined to be delivered on the R wave.

During ventricular fibrillation, the absence of an R wave determines the necessity of an asynchronous shock.

The high-energy pulse of short duration is delivered to the heart, thereby abolishing all cardiac electrical activity. The sinus node then takes over as the heart's rhythmical pacemaker.

Indications

1 Atrial flutter
2 Atrial fibrillation
3 Paroxysmal atrial tachycardia
4 Ventricular tachycardia
5 Ventricular fibrillation.

If cardioversion is indicated electively for atrial fibrillation, preliminary anticoagulation with warfarin for 2–3 weeks is necessary to reduce the risk of systemic embolism. Anticoagulation is advisable for 2 weeks after conversion until a stable sinus rhythm is assured.

If hypotension or bradycardia develops after cardioversion, administration of atropine and temporary pacing may be necessary.

Digitalis medication should be stopped for 48 hours before cardioversion is performed, as high digitalis levels may precipitate ventricular fibrillation or asystole during cardioversion. Cardioversion is also contraindicated if arrhythmias are the result of digitalis toxicity.

Method
The patient is anaesthetized and the electric pads are placed over the precordium. A shock of 50 J is administered at the predetermined peak of the R wave on the electrocardiogram.

The shock must not be given on the ascending limb of the T wave, as ventricular fibrillation may occur. If arrhythmia persists another shock at higher joules (100–200) may be necessary.

Further Reading
Barold, S. S., Mugica J. *The third decade of cardiac pacing. Advances in technology and clinical application.* Mt Kisco. New York: Futura Publishing Co. Inc., 1982.

Bolooki, H. *Clinical application of intra-aortic balloon pumping.* Mt Kisco. New York: Futura Publishing Co. Inc., 1977.

Chardack, W. M. Cardiac pacemakers and heart block: In: *Gibbon's surgery of the chest.* 3rd ed. Sabiston, D. C. and Spencer, F. C. (eds) Philadelphia: W. B. Saunders Co., 1976.

Kirklin, J. W., Barratt-Boyes, B. *Cardiac surgery.* New York: John Wiley and Sons, 1986.

Lowe, J. E., German, L. D. Cardiac Pacemakers. In: *Textbook of Surgery* 13th ed. Sabiston, D. C. Jr. (ed.) Philadelphia: W. B. Saunders Co., 1986.

Macoviak, J., Edmunds, L. H. Intra-aortic balloon pump – analysis of 5 years experience. *Ann. Thorac. Surg.* 29: 451, 1980.

Park, S. B., Lieber G. A., Burkholder, J. A. *et al.* Mechanical support of the failing heart. *Ann. Thorac. Surg.* 46: 627, 1986.

Sanfelippo, P. M., Baker, N. H., Ewy, H. G. *et al.* Experience with intra-aortic balloon counterpulsation. *Ann. Thorac. Surg.* 41: 36, 1986.

Smyth, N. P. D. Cardiac pacing. Collective Review. *Ann. Thorac. Surg.* 27: 270, 1979.

Zoll, P. M., Paul, M. H., Linenthal, A. J. *et al.* The effects of external electric currents on the heart: control of cardiac rhythm and induction and termination of cardiac arrhythmias. *Circulation* 14: 745, 1956.

Zumbro, G. L., Kitchens, W. R., Shearer, G. *et al.* Mechanical assistance for cardiogenic shock following cardiac surgery, myocardial infarction and cardiac transplantation. *Ann. Thorac. Surg.* 44: 11, 1987.

Chapter 3
Tachyarrhythmias

Normal sinus rhythm depends upon the inherent capacity of the conducting system of the heart to enjoy rhythmic spontaneous depolarization. As the cells in the sinoatrial node have the fastest inherent rhythmicity, this region serves as the heart's pacemaker, initiating waves of depolarization with spread across the atria to the atrioventricular node, through the bundle of His to reach the ventricles through the right and left bundle branches and its Purkinje fibres.

Sinus arrhythmia, with the heart speeding up during inspiration and slowing during expiration, is a normal occurrence in young people who have high vagal tone.

Sinus bradycardia and sinus tachycardia represent normal heart rates under 60 and over 100 per minute respectively, as the rate remains under the control of the sinoatrial node.

Arrhythmias
Cardiac rhythm wherein the impulse initiating the heart's contraction arises at a site other than the sinoatrial node:

Supraventricular arrhythmia
The pacemaker may be atrial or nodal (atrioventricular) causing:
1　Premature contractions
2　Paroxysmal tachycardias
3　Atrial flutter
4　Atrial fibrillation.

Ventricular arrhythmias
The pacemaker is in the ventricles causing:
1 Premature ventricular contractions
2 Ventricular tachycardia
3 Ventricular fibrillation.

Heart block
Atrioventricular block is represented by delay or total obstruction

of the passage of the sinoatrial impulse to the ventricles or at the level of the bundle of His or its branches. The causes include:

1 Drugs: quinidine, digitalis, propranolol, procainamide, excess potassium
2 Degenerative changes in the atrioventricular bundle: ischaemic heart disease; cardiac surgical trauma
3 Congenital anomalies of heart with heart block.

Re-entry tachycardia

A wave of electrical excitation is propagated in a circus movement within the myocardial syncitium.

1 Atrioventricular nodal re-entry tachycardia: there is a small circuit within the atrioventricular node
2 Wolff–Parkinson–White syndrome: the anomalous atrio-ventricular excitation is the result of a reciprocating tachycardia involving the A-V node, ventricular muscle, pathways and atrial muscle. The pre-excitation of part of the ventricle is reflected electrocardiographically by:

   a) Shortening of the P-R interval
   b) Widening of the QRS wave (delta wave)
   c) Secondary ST and T wave changes may result.

   The ventricular activation terminates at the normal time unless an associated bundle branch block is present.

Bundle of Kent

The presence of an accessory anomalous conduction pathway provides a shorter route to a portion of the ventricle than the normal junctional tissue, explaining the pre-excitation changes that cause re-entry tachycardias (Fig. 3.1).

Re-entry tachycardias may be initiated and terminated by appropriately timed stimuli administered during electrophysiological investigation with epicardial and endocardial mapping.

Although most tachyarrhythmias are amenable to medical management, surgical techniques have evolved for application when there is cardiac unresponsiveness to pharmacological management.

Surgical procedures
A-V node ablation with pacemaker insertion
Refractory supraventricular tachycardia can be managed by ablation
of the A-V node or the bundle of His combined with implantation
of a ventricular pacemaker (Fig. 3.2).

This procedure may be applicable to some cases of the WPW
syndrome where the reciprocating tachycardia uses the A-V node
as one limb of the tachycardia circuit.

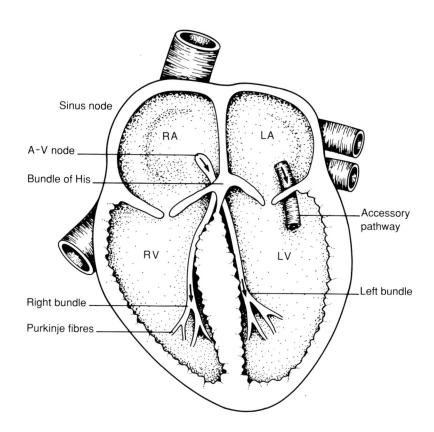

*Fig. 3.1. Diagrammatic representation of accessory anomalous conduction
pathway which bypasses the electrical insulation of the A-V groove,
allowing early ventricular excitation of part of the ventricles.*

Ventricular aneurysmectomy with removal of excitable zones
Electrophysiological mapping may indicate the associated need
for either encircling endocardial ventriculotomy or endocardial
resection.

Division of accessory pathways
This procedure is specifically applicable in the Wolff–Parkinson–
White syndrome. Although most patients with this condition are
asymptomatic, some present with two possible patterns of
arrhythmia.

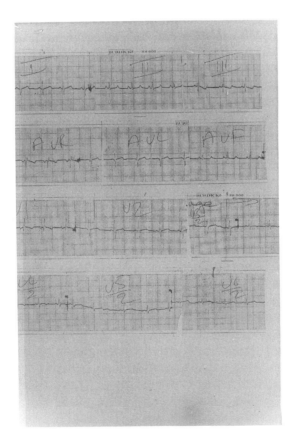

Fig 3.2. ECG of patient after A-V node ablation and pacemaker implantation.

1 Reciprocating tachycardia with antegrade conduction over the
   A-V node with return of conduction to the atria via the accessory
   pathway.
2 Atrial fibrillation with rapid ventricular response due to the
   conduction along the accessory pathway, bypassing the A-V
   node and its customary refractory period. Medical management of these arrhythmias is often successful, but failure of
   response or non-compliance may provide justification for
   surgical measures.

Surgical techniques

The operation is a highly specialized one utilizing cardiopulmonary
bypass. As the atrioventricular connections may be anywhere on
the A-V ring, preliminary study of electrocardiographic patterns
and endocardial catheter mapping are necessary to establish the
exact location of the conducting pathways.

The location is confirmed at operation by epicardial mapping
with division of the accessory pathways. A good result can be
anticipated if the pathway is located in the right free wall of the
heart.

Pathways along the left free wall which are close to the coronary
sinus or the circumflex coronary artery are less likely to give good
results.

Ablation of the pathway may be done by sharp dissection and
division or by cryosurgical methods.

The combination of electrophysiological study and understanding of the mechanisms and anatomical basis of certain
arrhythmias determines the success of the well planned surgical
procedures, which may vary from simple ventriculotomy, division
of bundle branches to local ablation.

Further Reading

Harrison L., Gallagher J. J. et al. Cryosurgical ablation of the AV node His
    bundle: A new method for producing AV block. *Circulation* 55:464, 1977.
Josephson M. E., Harken A. H., Horowitz L. N. Endocardial excision – a
    new surgical technique for the treatment of recurrent ventricular
    tachycardia. *Circulation* 60:1430, 1979.

Sealy W. C., Wallace A. G. Surgical treatment of Wolff–Parkinson–White syndrome. *J. Thorac. Cardiovasc. Surg.* 68:757, 1974.

Sealy W. C., Miket E. M. Anatomical problems with identification and interruption of posterior septal Kent bundles. *Ann. Thorac. Surg.* 32:429, 1981.

Sealy W. C., Gallagher J. J., Kasell J. H. His bundle interruption for control of inappropriate ventricular response to atrial arrhythmias. *Ann. Thorac. Surg.* 32:429, 1981.

Chapter 4
Cardiovascular Trauma

Injuries to the heart and associated thoracic structures may be due to:

1 *Blunt non-penetrating trauma*
   a) Acceleration injury: pedestrian struck by car
   b) Deceleration injury: car or aeroplane passengers
   c) Crushing injury: weight falling on chest

2 *Penetrating trauma*
Gunshot wound; stabbing injury; cardiac surgery; perforation by cardiac catheter.

Associated injuries may affect the lungs, tracheobronchial airway system, oesophagus, diaphragm and great vessels. Investigative assessment of such potential structural damage will require appropriate attention.

Cardiac trauma

1 Myocardial contusion, laceration or damage to coronary arteries may precipitate myocardial infarction. Proper monitoring of such patients in the coronary care unit with study of enzymes and electrocardiogram is essential for several days.
2 Ventricular septum may suffer perforation with development of a septal defect and its clinical effects.
3 Valves: rupture of valve cusps or papillary muscles, with special predilection for the aortic valve, will lead to the development of valvular incompetence.
4 Conduction disturbances: the development of heart block and other arrhythmias will need special attention to avoid sudden death due to ventricular fibrillation.
5 Cardiac tamponade: haemopericardium leads to compression of the heart with poor ventricular filling during diastole. Clinical features include elevated jugular vein pressure, fall in systemic blood pressure and pulsus paradoxus – the pulse amplitude paradoxically increasing during inspiration. Cyanosis and signs of cardiogenic shock will proceed to death.

Pericardiocentesis may provide temporary relief of cardiac tamponade and is carried out while intravenous infusions, endotracheal intubation and other diagnostic and therapeutic measures are started.

Definitive repair of the underlying cardiac injury requires sternotomy, removal of blood from the pericardial cavity and control of bleeding by digital compression.

Right atrial and right ventricular stab wounds can usually be repaired with pledgeted sutures without need for cardio-pulmonary bypass, which should always be on standby readiness. Most other cardiac injuries will require extracorporeal circulation facilities.

Aortic trauma

The aortic wall consists of intima, media and adventitia. The media, which supplies elasticity by virtue of its smooth muscle and elastic tissue, does not provide great tensile strength but the adventitia with its fibrous tissue content provides 60% of the aorta's tensile strength and can resist intraluminal pressure of 1000 mmHg before bursting.

Injury to the great vessels is a cause of high mortality. Death may ensue because of exsanguination or from compression of vital structures by internal haemorrhage.

Rupture of the aorta is most commonly the result of an automobile accident. It represents a sudden deceleration effect with shearing forces affecting three major immobile or fixed areas of the thoracic aorta, where a sudden rise in intraluminal pressure tears the aorta while the remainder of the mobile aorta is carried forward by the momentum of its contained blood.

1 At the aortic root: the most common aortic tear occurs above the aortic valve with haemorrhage within the pericardium causing instantaneous death from tamponade.

2 At the aortic isthmus: at the site of the ligamentum arteriosum just beyond the subclavian artery; 80% of these patients will die immediately at the scene of the accident from exsanguination. 10–15% will survive for about 8 hours as the blood is contained within the adventitia.

A high index of suspicion regarding this diagnosis is essential, especially where a steering wheel injury to the sternum has occurred. Clinical features include dyspnoea, back pain and differences between upper limb pulses. The presence of widening of the mediastinum on chest radiograms makes immediate aortography mandatory. Once the condition is diagnosed, immediate operation is indicated (Fig. 4.1).

In a small percentage of cases a traumatic aneurysm may develop, encased by peri-haematoma fibrosis as a false aneurysm, and present clinically months or years after the accident.

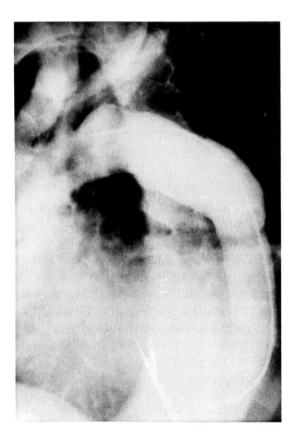

Fig. 4.1. Aortographic view of aortic rupture.

3 At the diaphragmatic hiatus: as soon as a diagnosis of aortic rupture is made operation is carried out, with proximal and distal control of the aorta established before dissecting the area of tear with its haematoma. Repair may require interposition of a dacron tube graft if the two ends of the aorta cannot be approximated.

Further Reading

Akins C. W., Buckley M. J., Dagget W. *et al.* Acute traumatic disruption of the thoracic aorta: A ten year experience. *Ann. Thorac. Surg.* 31: 305, 1981.

Arom K. V., Richardson J. D. *et al.* Subxiphoid pericardial window in patients with suspected traumatic pericardial tamponade. *Ann. Thorac. Surg.* 23, 545, 1977.

Mandal A. K., Awariefe S. O., Oparah S. S. Experience in the management of 50 consecutive penetrating wounds of the heart. *Br. J. Surg.* 66: 565, 1979.

McBride L. R., Tidik S. Sothert J. C. *et al.* Primary repair of traumatic aortic disruption. *Ann. Thorac. Surg.* 43; 65, 1987.

Symbas A. M. Penetrating cardiac wounds: A comparison of different therapeutic methods. *Ann. Thorac. Surg.* 183: 377, 1976.

Trinkle J. K., Grover F. L. *The management of thoracic trauma victims.* Philadelphia: J. B. Lippincott, 1980.

Chapter 5
Cardiopulmonary Bypass

The essential determinants for cardiac surgical success include a comprehensive preoperative assessment of the patient, accurate definition of the fundamental lesion and ameliorative treatment of secondary effects such as cardiac failure, electrolyte imbalance and arrhythmia.

In addition to the application of technical expertise in the performance of specific operative procedures, an optimal outcome depends upon good intra-operative anaesthetic management, the efficient collaboration of pump technicians and dedicated intensive care management in the postoperative period.

Preparation for operation

The presence of a technically correctable cardiac lesion is best treated surgically before myocardial decompensation materially increases the risk of operative mortality and the probability of postoperative morbidity.

A thorough history and physical examination with urinalysis, blood count, haematocrit, electrocardiogram, chest radiography and echocardiography are essential.

Patients who have been on digitalis and diuretics must be evaluated regarding serum electrolytes and renal function, with notation of serum creatinine and urea–nitrogen levels.

Irreversible damage to other systems, e.g. kidneys, liver or lungs provides a contraindication to operative correction of the lesion because of the high fatality rate.

Careful preoperative analysis of echocardigraphic details and, if indicated, cardiac catheterization results and angiocardiographic data, permits an accurate diagnosis of anatomic abnormalities and physiological derangements.

The blood bank is alerted regarding the amount of blood, plasma, platelets and other components that may be required for each patient. Digitalis therapy may need to be continued up to the time of surgery if rapid fibrillation or congestive heart failure be present, but ideally should be stopped 24 hours prior to operation. Diuretics are stopped 48 hours before operation. If the patient is receiving more than 160 mg propranolol per day, dosage reduction for several days before operation is recommended. Coumarin is discontinued 48 hours before operation and prothrombin time checked.

Preoperative dental evaluation is essential in patients who are to undergo valve replacement, aortic grafting or the intracardiac placement of prosthetic material. All patients undergoing cardiac surgical procedures will have prophylactic antibiotic cover. Intravenous antibiosis is initiated in the operating theatre and continues until all central lines, chest tubes and Foley catheters have been removed. If antibiotic therapy is continued for longer than 48 hours, then daily culture of sputum, blood and urine should be carried out in case resistant organisms develop. Amendments in type of antibiotic or dosage may be necessary if renal dysfunction is present.

Historic highlights

Although Rehn of Frankfurt first successfully repaired a cardiac stab wound, it was Souttar's successful digital dilatation of the mitral valve in 1925 that declared a new era. The successful ligation of a patent ductus arteriosus by Robert Gross in 1938, and his later successful resection of an aortic coarctation in 1944, also independently carried out by Crafoord in that year, heralded new horizons. In the same year Alfred Blalock and Helen Taussig introduced the subclavian–pulmonary shunt for tetralogy of Fallot, with conversion of cyanotic heart disease to a palliative acyanotic state. The resurrection of digital dilatation of the mitral valve in 1948 by Brock in London and Bailey in Philadelphia, and the introduction of hypothermia by Bigelow in Toronto in that year, finally culminated in the introduction of cardiopulmonary bypass for closure of an atrial septal defect by Gibbon in 1953.

Cardiopulmonary bypass for cardiac surgery

The establishment of an extracorporeal circulation by cardio-pulmonary bypass represents the greatest single innovative advance in cardiac surgery. It is a technique whereby the pumping action of the heart and the gas-exchange functions of the lung are temporarily replaced by a mechanical device, the pump oxygenator, attached to the patient's cardiovascular system.

It is an essential prerequisite for all types of intracardiac procedures, coronary revascularization and operations on the thoracic aorta.

Partial temporary cardiopulmonary bypass with a membrane oxygenator has also been utilized in children with severe reversible respiratory distress.

Pathophysiological effects of cardiopulmonary bypass
The cardiopulmonary device must be capable of receiving up to 6 l of venous blood per minute, spreading it into a thin film prior to exposure to oxygen. After exchange of oxygen and carbon dioxide, the blood is infused under pressure by a roller-pump mechanism into the patient's arterial system without damaging the blood components and without introducing air emboli. Inevitable changes in the patient's own blood flow, blood pressure and intravascular volume, as well as changes in pH and electrolyte content, need to be monitored and remedied.

Adverse effects
1 *Blood damage*: Haemolysis, denaturation of proteins and microembolism with aggregated red cells, air, fibrin and fat become possible with prolonged bypass. Thrombocytopenia, reduction of clotting factors and fibrinolysis may develop. The delayed development of a normochromic, normocytic anaemia is not unusual.
2 *Changes in pulmonary function*: Patchy alveolar atelectasis with diminished pulmonary compliance may develop 24–48 hours after bypass, with shunting of unoxygenated blood through the underventilated alveoli resulting in a ventilation–perfusion derangement with resulting hypoxia.
3 *Electrolyte disturbances*: If the perfusate is primed with Dextrose or Mannitol, the ensuing diuresis may aggravate the loss of potassium during cardiopulmonary bypass, with the development of serious arrhythmias.
4 *Acid–base changes*: Inadequate oxygenation during bypass may cause tissue anoxia, with the development of metabolic acidosis and subsequent depression of myocardial contractility.

Technical manoeuvres

A median sternotomy provides ideal access to the heart, ascending aorta and large venous channels for appropriate cannulation so that blood is removed from the venous system by gravity and flows to the oxygenator, which has within it a heat exchanger and reservoir from where it is pumped into the arterial system.

The patient is heparinized and a haemochron is used to monitor the activated clotting time (ACT) which should be kept above 450s so that the extracorporeal system does not clot.

1 *Arterial cannulation*: Two concentric purse-string sutures of 3-0 dexxon are placed in the aortic adventitia and media at the aortic site of election just before the origin of the innominate artery. A small stab wound into the aortic lumen provides entry for a tapered aortic cannula, which is then secured by tourniquet control. The cannula is connected to the arterial line after assurance that all air bubbles have been removed from the system.

   The ilio-femoral artery may be preferred for arterial return in operations on the aortic arch, and in some cases of "redo" aorto-coronary bypass procedures.

2 *Venous cannulation*: Systemic venous blood flow to the pump oxygenator may be attained by a single large right atrial cannula inserted through the atrial appendage, or via two vena caval cannulae joined by a Y-connector. A single atrial catheter is suitable for most aortocoronary bypass procedures and for aortic valve replacement. Caval cannulae are necessary for repair of most congenital intracardiac defects and for procedures on the mitral, tricuspid and pulmonary valves.

   Total bypass is attained by encircling the intrapericardial segments of both venae cavae with tape-snares, which are tightened to compress the caval walls against the cannulae, directing all the venous blood to the oxygenator (Fig. 5.1).

   A persistent left superior vena cava must be separately cannulated through the right atrium and coronary sinus to prevent blood flooding the operative field.

   Coronary sinus blood is removed by suction through the opened right atrium or by venting the left ventricle by inserting a venting cannula into the superior pulmonary vein and manipulating it into the left ventricle. The left ventricle can also be vented directly at its apex, returning bronchial venous blood being controlled. Venting may also be accomplished effectively via the main pulmonary artery.

3   *Intracardiac suction*
   a) Venting catheter: gentle suction on the venting catheter is applied by a separate occlusive pump which adds to the venous return and decompresses the heart.
   b) Intracardiac sucker: a separate occlusive pump aspirates blood from the opened heart. Any debris is trapped in a miniport filter interposed between the suction line and the oxygenator.

Oxygenators

Venous blood may be oxygenated and carbon dioxide removed in the extracorporeal circulation in three possible ways:

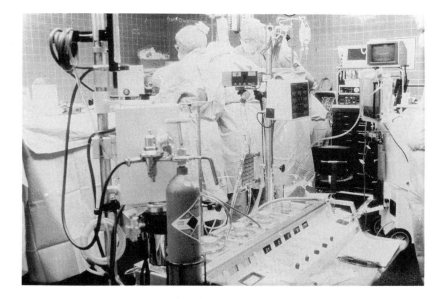

Fig. 5.1. Extracorporeal pump oxygenator in use during open heart operative procedure.

1 *Disposable bubble oxygenator*: After oxygenation of the venous blood is attained by bubbles of oxygen, the froth has to be defoamed with silicone. Any residual bubbles are eliminated in the defoaming section of the mechanical device by a surface-tension reducing agent. This comprises a quantity of open-cell polyurethane foam treated with silicone antifoam enclosed in a knitted dacron sleeve with a pore size of 120 μm. Here the bubbles coalesce and are removed from the blood which now passes to the arterial reservoir at the base of the oxygenating chamber.

2 *Screen oxygenator*: A thin film of blood passes through an atmosphere of oxygen on a screen, which may be still or rotating.

3 *Membrane oxygenator*: Blood and oxygen are separated by a thin permeable membrane. A closed polyvinyl chloride (PVC) reservoir receives the venous blood which is pumped through the membrane oxygenator. A semipermeable membrane is interposed between the blood and oxygenating gas. The Saarns membrane oxygenator consists of a polypropylene membrane with a pore size 200–400A, which is supported on a mesh and closely welded on a spacer into a compact format and enclosed in a rigid plastic casing. There are separate channels for blood and gas.

Membrane oxygenators cause less destruction to formed elements with maintenance of platelet function. Gaseous micro-emboli are uncommon, permitting long-term extracorporeal support and utilization in infants with respiratory distress syndrome.

Arterial pumps

The roller pump is generally used to return blood from the oxygenator to the patient and to provide power suction for aspiration of intracardiac and pericardiac blood.

Compliant silastic tubing is inserted into the roller pumps, which are gently occlusive. Flow rates are established by the revolution rate of the pump. Modern roller pumps have low-inertia pump heads and a large stepping motor which, when used in conjunction with a control module, can accelerate and decelerate intermittently to produce a pulsatile flow at conventional flow rates and with a pulse pressure in excess of 30 mmHg.

Pulsatile perfusion is associated with lower levels of peripheral vascular resistance during bypass. This permits better tissue perfusion with demonstrable benefit to renal, cerebral and pancreatic function. There is also reduced left ventricular afterload at the end of perfusion, probably due to lower level of plasma angiotension II.

Arterial blood pressure
During cardiopulmonary bypass in normothermic or mildly hypothermic adults, the mean arterial pressure should not be permitted to fall below 55 mmHg for any prolonged period. Reduced cerebral blood flow may increase the incidence of subsequent cerebral complications, while diminished renal blood flow will lead to anuria. Inotropic agents such as dopamine or dobutamine may be required to maintain the mean arterial pressure above 70 mmHg.

If arterial blood pressure rises to high levels with a mean over 100 mmHg, the risk of cerebral haemorrhage is sufficiently great to justify the use of vasodilating agents such as nitroprusside (nipride) to lower the blood pressure.

Temperature
The introduction of hypothermia in patients during extracorporeal bypass reduces oxygen consumption, thereby permitting tissues to survive longer periods of poor or no perfusion. The safety of periods of circulatory arrest or low flow is inversely related to the patient's temperature. A level of 28°C provides the optimal milieu, should temporary mechanical failure occur during extracorporeal support. This temperature level also improves operating conditions if reduction or cessation of perfusion is required temporarily.

Heat exchangers
Cooling and warming of patients during cardiopulmonary bypass is done with an efficient heat exchanger, which is an integral part of the oxygenator. It is occasionally necessary to cool infants under 2 years of age, as an initial step, with ice-bags to about 30°C.

The heat exchanger receives water from a thermostatically controlled mixing valve which is used to induce and reverse systemic hypothermia.

It is advisable to exceed a gradient greater than 15°C between the arterial line temperature and the patient's nasopharyngeal temperature. Similarly, during rewarming the blood is warmed to no greater than 15°C above the patient's temperature in order to minimize the formation of bubbles in the blood as the solubility of gas decreases with the rise in temperature.

Anticoagulation

Extracorporeal circulation requires adequate anticoagulation. The dosage of heparin required to induce such anticoagulation during open heart surgery is best guided by frequent assay of activated clotting time. A priming dose of 3–4 mg/kg of heparin is administered intravenously prior to cardiac cannulation and after baseline measurement of ACT. ACT levels are monitored at 30 minute intervals during bypass and maintained by additive heparin administration, if necessary, to maintain an ACT greater than 450s.

Protamine

On completion of bypass and removal of the venous cannulae, with the aortic cannula still in place, protamine is given intravenously in a dose of 1.3 mg per mg of heparin, after which the cardiotomy suckers should not be used, lest coagulation of blood occurs in the oxygenator. Added protamine may be necessary to bring the ACT to the desired postoperative level.

Prolonged bleeding, despite a normal ACT and adequate vascular integrity, implies platelet dysfunction and should be treated with infusion of platelet concentrate, even though the platelet count is within normal limits.

Continued bleeding: Other reasons may be:
1 Dilution of clotting factors
2 Consumptive coagulopathy
3 Increased fibrinolytic activity
4 Heparin- or protamine-induced coagulopathy
5 Destruction of platelets: prostacyclin, now available for use

during open heart surgery, is synthesized by intact endo-
theliac surfaces and protects platelets during exposure to a
foreign surface.

Cardiotomy reservoirs

During the extracorporeal circulation, blood from the cardiac
cavities passes through a cardiotomy reservoir prior to flowing
into the oxygenator. The cardiotomy reservoir also contains
defoamers and filters, thereby removing formed blood elements,
blood clots, fat globules and debris from diseased valves.

All tubing and connectors used during bypass must be
presterilized. Polyvinyl chloride (PVC) tubing presterilized with
ethylene oxide is used to connect the various machine components
to each other and to the patient.

The various components are assembled by the perfusionist,
with the arterial and venous circuit in continuity with the pump-
oxygenator circuit. The machine is primed and the priming fluid
circulated through the apparatus via the arteriovenous loop circuit
at an operative flow rate. Suckers and left ventricular vent are
similarly connected to the circuit.

The arteriovenous loop is then clamped and divided by the
surgeon and appropriate ends of the tube are connected to the
arterial and venous cannulae after all air bubbles have been
eliminated from the circuit. Perfusion can now commence.

Priming fluids

The pump-oxygenator system needs to be primed with a volume
of perfusate appropriate to the patient's size. In an adult 2–3 l of
priming fluid are necessary, with significantly smaller volumes for
children. Although blood represents the ideal perfusate, logistic
demands on blood banks, the risk of transfusion hepatitis, iso-
antibody formation and allergic reactions, has fostered the haemodilution techniques for cardiopulmonary bypass.

Haemodilution using crystalloid solutions such as 5% dextrose,
or balanced salt solutions such as plasmalyte and mannitol has the
advantage of stimulating larger urine flows during and after bypass.
There is a reduced incidence of platelet aggregate embolization
and a reduction in systemic vascular resistance.

As blood temperature drops, there is increased viscosity of the perfusate with reduced oxygen-carrying capacity due to haemodilution. This can be compensated during bypass by increasing the blood flow rate. During hypothermia tissue oxygen consumption falls to 50% of normal at 30°C and to 20% of normal at 20°C.

Myocardial protection
Cold cardioplegic solutions have demonstrably served to protect and preserve the myocardium during the operative cardiac procedures, while extracorporeal circulation is maintained by the pump oxygenator and the aorta is cross-clamped.

A good cardioplegic solution causes immediate cardiac arrest with conservation of intracellular substrates. It maintains cellular integrity for a prolonged period.

Myocardial cooling to 20°C minimizes anaerobic metabolism, permitting longer periods of myocardial ischemia. Cardioplegia produces a flaccid motionless heart. The bloodless operative field that is created aids the performance of expeditious surgical manoeuvres and permits repair of complex cardiac lesions.

Current cardioplegic techniques utilize either pure crystalloid cardioplegia or blood cardioplegia with a 4 to 1 admixture of crystalloid and pump blood which, some claim, reduces reperfusion cardiac injury.

Current cold cardioplegic technique utilizes a mixture of 500 ml 5% dextrose and 0.5% sodium chloride at a temperature of 6°C. To this fluid is added 20 mM potassium chloride (1492 mg); 7.5 mM magnesium chloride (1527 mg); 1 mM calcium chloride (147 mg) and 2.5 mM bicarbonate ion (210mg).

In an adult the injection of 500 ml, at mildly hypothermic levels, into the aortic root will maintain asystole up to 1 hour. Topical cold lactated Ringer's solution may also be poured over the epicardial surface of the heart to maintain generalized cardiac hypothermia.

In procedures for aortic valve replacement, after the aortotomy has been accomplished, special mushroom-tipped catheters may be inserted directly into the coronary ostia and 200 ml of cold cardioplegic solution infused directly into each coronary artery.

Monitoring during open heart surgery
Maintenance of the patient's homeostasis during extracorporeal circulation requires comprehensive monitoring of vital functions before, during and after open heart surgery. During extracorporeal support a blood-flow rate of 2.4 l/m/min provides adequate tissue perfusion. Inadequate tissue perfusion is reflected in the development of metabolic acidosis with hyperkalaemia and diminished urinary output.

The monitoring console records and displays arterial as well as right and left atrial pressures, a continuous electrocardiographic pattern and oesophageal temperature. The urinary output is monitored.

Frequent measurement of blood gases, pH, acid–base status, haemoglobin and packed-cell volume, plasma sodium and potassium levels, ACT and serum osmolality, are carried out and recorded.

A fibrillator and a synchronous R-wave defibrillator should be available.

After discontinuation of cardiopulmonary bypass, any aberrations in levels of haemoglobin, potassium level, pH and base deficit should be remedied. Cardiac arrhythmia and hypotension may need appropriate therapy.

Decannulation
This process involves a reversal of the procedures used in establishing extracorporeal circulation. The prevention of air embolism is first accomplished by evacuation of air from the multiple recesses of the left ventricle, left atrial appendage and pulmonary veins. Air may be trapped for long periods despite good cardiac output, with devastating delayed effects. After completion of the intracardiac procedures and when the heart or aorta is closed, the cardiac chambers are permitted to fill with blood and as the left ventricle begins to eject with the aortic clamp still in place, a needle is placed into the ascending aorta and air evacuated through it. With the patient in the head-down position, the aortic clamp is released while the anaesthetist inflates the lungs with positive pressure.

Once all air has been evacuated, utilizing the aortic vent, the left ventricular vent and massage of the heart chambers, full perfusion flow is re-established. The patient is gradually rewarmed, while appropriate support of the circulating blood volume and systemic pressure is carried out and any required pharmacological support provided. Re-institution of partial bypass may be necessary to provide temporary mechanical support. Acid–base, electrolyte and blood gas status are corrected if necessary.

Once satisfactory spontaneous cardiac activity is established decannulation proceeds. The left ventricular vent is removed and the purse-string suture tied. Pacemaker electrodes are sutured to the heart and exteriorized. Bypass is gradually terminated and the venous lines are clamped and removed. Protamine is slowly administered to neutralize the residual heparin effect. The aortic cannula is the last to be removed, blood being administered through it from the pump-oxygenator if required.

Final assessment is made of all cardiac and anastomotic suture lines and preparation made for closure of the sternotomy wound, with placement of a mediastinal tube drain which is exteriorized.

Complications of cardiopulmonary bypass
1 *Mechanical*: Electrical, mechanical or oxygenator failure is prevented by good maintenance and care of the equipment.
2 *Air embolism* from the arterial line or vent is
   a) A preventable complication due to inadequate removal of air after cardiotomy
   b) Perfusionist error: emptying of oxygenator arterial reservoir, defective oxygenator, detachment of oxygenator during bypass, reversal of pump tubing or reversed direction of pump rotation.

Unexpected ventricular contraction with the aorta unclamped may be a source of air embolism but is prevented by the presence of a vent.

Postoperative management
Among the postoperative sequalae that must be anticipated and monitored are:

1 Cardiac: low output syndrome; congestive failure; arrhythmias; cardiac tamponade
2 Haemorrhage: assess whether re-exploration of mediastinum is necessary or whether coagulation disorders need treatment
3 Renal failure
4 Pulmonary insufficiency
5 Disorders of acid–base balance
6 Hepatic dysfunction and jaundice.

Endotracheal intubation is maintained for 24 hours, with appropriate ventilatory support. Bronchial suction, intermittent positive pressure breathing, aerosol and physiotherapy may be required.

Alterations in acid–base balance are remedied, with administration of bicarbonate to remedy acidosis.

Continued postoperative measurement of right and left atrial pressure, and continuous electrocardiographic monitoring, are essential. Administration of diuretics, digitalis, vasopressor or inotropic agents, and anti-arrhythmic drugs may be indicated. Maintenance of good cardiac output may require Isoprenaline and attachment of pacer wires to a portable generator may be necessary. Dobutamine and calcium may need to be administered.

Antibiotic administration commenced intraoperatively is continued until all catheters and tubes are removed.

Good urinary output is maintained by adequate blood and fluid administration and use of frusemide and mannitol.

Blood losses from the retrosternal spaces are recorded and replaced by blood transfusion if indicated.

A chest X-ray is performed immediately on return to the recovery room, 6 hours later, and the following morning.

Blood gases are monitored hourly for 4 hours postoperatively, then 2 hourly for 4 hours, then 4 hourly for 24 hours.

Haemoglobin, haematocrit and platelet count are checked at 1 hour, 6 hours and 24 hours after operation. Electrolytes are similarly checked 2 hourly for 6 hours, then 6 hourly for 24 hours postoperatively.

Summary

Extracorporeal cardiopulmonary bypass is a prerequisite for successful open heart operations. It is now a routine procedure, the success of whose performance is dependent on the integration and collaboration of surgeons, anaesthetists, perfusionists and nursing personnel utilizing the complementary services of laboratory and associated technicians. It is a team effort whose final reward is a satisfactory patient outcome.

Postoperative low cardiac output

1 *Myocardial infarction*: Confirmed by electrocardiography and serum enzymes.
2 *Cardiac tamponade*: Requires evacuation of blood
3 *Inadequate atrial filling*: Requires fluid volume
4 *Depressed myocardial contractility*
   a) High filling pressure: requires Dobutamine (Beta agonist)
   b) Low cardiac index: vasodilator therapy (nipride) balloon counterpulsation.

Further Reading

Barratt-Boyes B. G., Simpson M., Neutze J. M. Intracardiac surgery in neonates and infants using deep hypothermia with surface cooling and limited cardiopulmonary bypass. *Circulation* 43: 25, 1971.

Gibbon J. H. Application of a mechanical heart and lung apparatus to cardiac surgery. *Minn. Med.* 37: 171, 1954.

Ionescu M. I. *Techniques in extracorporeal circulation.* 2nd ed. Butterworths. London. 1981.

Kirklin J. W., Barratt-Boyes B. G. *Cardiac surgery.* John Wiley and Sons. New York. 1986.

Kirklin H. K., Blackstone E. H., Kirklin J. W. Cardiopulmonary bypass: studies on its damaging effects. *Blood Purif.* 5: 168, 1987.

Utley J. R., Betleski R. *Pathophysiology and techniques of cardiopulmonary bypass.* Vol. II. Williams and Wilkins. Baltimore. 1983.

PART II
ACQUIRED HEART DISEASE

Chapter 6
Pericarditis

Acute pericarditis
As the pericardium is a closed sac enveloping the heart, inflammation of the pericardium is usually accompanied by a small pericardial effusion.

Aetiology
1 *Infective*:
   a) Viral pericarditis is common and may be due to Coxsackie, influenzal or other viruses
   b) Pyogenic: due to streptococcal, staphylococcal or *Haemophilus influenzae* infection. Infection may complicate cardiac catheterization or insertion of pacing electrodes
   c) Tuberculous spread to the pericardium from infected mediastinal lymph nodes
   d) Mycotic infection may cause pericarditis.
2 *Myocardial infarction* may cause a localized pericarditis over the infarct but at times generalized pericarditis may occur.
3 *Uraemic pericarditis* develops frequently in patients with end stage renal disease maintained on dialysis.
4 *Connective tissue diseases*: Pericarditis is a frequent concomitant in rheumatic fever, systemic lupus and polyarteritis nodosa.
5 *Neoplastic pericardial effusion* due to invasion by bronchogenic carcinoma or metastatic spread from breast or elsewhere.
6 *Traumatic pericarditis*: Thoracic trauma, recent cardiac surgery (Tressier's post-cardiotomy or Dressler's syndrome) or radiation therapy to chest.

Clinical features
After a prodromal few days of fever, malaise, perspiration and a dry cough, there is an acute development of a sharp precordial pain aggravated by breathing, coughing or swallowing.

A pericardial "to and fro" friction rub is audible on auscultation until a large pericardial effusion develops, when the friction rub disappears.

41

Radiological examination demonstrates a globular enlargement of the cardiac silhouette. (Fig. 6.1).

Electrocardiography may demonstrate ST elevation with later T wave flattening or depression.

Echocardiography and CT scan of the thorax will demonstrate the pericardial effusion.

In the presence of a pericardial effusion the development of cardiac tamponade will cause distension of neck veins, hepatomegaly with ascites, and pulsus paradoxus. Cardiac arrhythmias may develop.

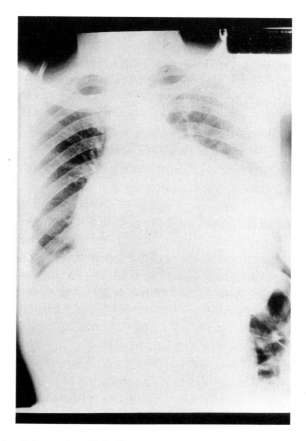

Fig. 6.1. Pericardial effusion demonstrated radiologically.

Treatment
Antibiotics, an anti-tuberculous regime or chemotherapy will be indicated for infective, tuberculous or malignant disease respectively. Prednisone is indicated in viral pericarditis. Increased frequency of dialysis may be necessary in uraemic pericarditis.

Evacuation of pericardial effusion
1 *Pericardiocentesis*
   Aspiration of a pericardial effusion may be an emergency procedure in tamponade due to a traumatic haemopericardium. It may need to be done urgently when cardiac embarrassment is due to an enlarging pericardial effusion. It may be an elective diagnostic procedure to provide a sample of pericardial fluid.
   Needle aspiration may be done under local anaesthesia via three alternative routes:
   a) Xiphisternally: the needle is introduced to the left of the xiphoid at the xipho-costal angle and angled at 45° to the horizontal and 45° to the midline and directed towards the left axilla.
   b) Apically: the needle is introduced at the apex and directed at 45° to the horizontal or directed towards the right scapula.
   c) Left parasternally in the 5th interspace.
   The risk of penetrating the myocardium via any of these routes can be reduced by attaching the needle to lead V of an electrocardiograph. ST segment deviation will indicate that the myocardium has been penetrated. The needle should then be withdrawn slightly into the pericardial sac.
2 *Pericardiostomy*
   a) Subxiphoid: under local anaesthesia a 7 cm midline incision is centred over the xiphoid. The tissues are dissected until the anterior–inferior aspect of the pericardium is visualized. A biopsy specimen of pericardium is excised without endangering the coronary vessels. The pericardial fluid is evacuated and a tube appropriately placed for continuous drainage and, if necessary, antibiotic instillation.
   b) Parasternal: under general anaesthesia the left 5th costal cartilage is resected. A pericardial biopsy is taken without penetrating the pleura and a drainage tube is placed.

c) Pericardial window: through a left 6th interspace thoracotomy, a window of pericardium is resected permitting continued pericardial drainage to empty into the left pleural cavity, which is drained to an underwater seal by a thoracostomy tube. This procedure is especially indicated in uraemic pericarditis.

Constrictive pericarditis

The heart becomes enveloped by dense, rigid pericardial fibrosis, which often becomes secondarily calcified. The chronic constrictive process develops slowly over several years following tuberculous pericarditis. Rarely it may complicate pneumococcal pericarditis. The condition leads to restriction of diastolic filling of the heart, thereby reducing stroke volume and cardiac output.

Clinical features

Characteristically right heart failure with distended neck veins, hepatomegaly and ascites provide the usual manifestations. Liver functions are impaired.

Arterial pressure tends to be low with diminished pulse pressure. Pulsus paradoxus is notable. Examination of the heart demonstrates a small quiet impulse with distant heart sounds.

Radiological chest examination usually suggests a normal heart size with clear lung fields. Calcification may be noted. Fluoroscopy shows impaired or absent heart pulsation.

Electrocardiography reveals a normal sinus rhythm with low voltage and broad and notched P waves. Atrial fibrillation may be demonstrated.

Echocardiography will demonstrate the fibrotic, constrictive pericardial tissue.

Cardiac catheterization is rarely indicated in this condition. A typical right ventricular pressure pattern displays an early dip at the onset of diastole followed by an abrupt and early rise to an elevated plateau throughout diastole. Right atrial pressure is sustained at a high level.

Surgical treatment

Decortication of the heart is a definitive procedure that removes the chronically inflamed, thickened and fibrotic constrictive pericardium which limits diastolic filling.

A midline sternotomy provides ample exposure of both ventricles, great vessels and the right atrium.

Although cardiopulmonary bypass is rarely necessary it should be readily available.

An incision is made through the thickened pericardium over the right ventricle. With auxiliary cruciate incisions, planes of cleavage are developed to permit flaps of pericardium to be dissected from the underlying right and left ventricles.

Decortication of the thin-walled right atrium is done with care, any lacerations being repaired with pledgeted prolene sutures.

The phrenic nerves and its vessels are preserved and care is taken not to damage the coronary vessels, with special attention to the right coronary artery in the atrioventricular groove.

Further Reading

Darsee J. R., Braunwald E. Diseases of the pericardium. In: Braunwald E. (Ed.), *Heart disease: A textbook of cardiovascular medicine.* W. B. Saunders Co. Philadelphia. 1980.

Dressler W. The post myocardial infarction syndrome: A report of 44 cases. *A. A. A. Arch. Int. Med.* 102: 23, 1989.

Miller J., Mansour K., Hatcher C. Pericardiectomy: Current indications, concepts and results in a university center. *Ann. Thorac. Surg.* 34: 40, 1980.

Prager R., Wilson C., Bender H. The subxiphoid approach to pericardial disease. *Ann. Thorac. Surg.* 34: 6, 1982.

Tajik A. J. Echocardiography in pericardial effusion. *Am. J. Med.* 63: 29, 1977.

Chapter 7
Bacterial Endocarditis

Acute bacterial endocarditis results from the bacterial invasion of a heart valve or an area of endocardium. It may develop during a bout of acute septicaemia, with a virulent organism such as *Streptococcus pyogenes, Staphylococcus aureus* or *Neisseria gonococcus* invading a previously normal heart valve and destroying it.

The condition is associated with overwhelming infection in drug addicts, immunosuppressed individuals and in infants under 2 years of age.

Blood cultures reveal the nature of the organisms, while 2-D echocardiography will define the valvular destruction and vegetations on the valve cusps.

Marantic endocarditis is a form of acute bacterial endocarditis that develops in patients with terminal cancer.

Subacute bacterial endocarditis

The conditions results from a bacteraemia that is precipitated by dental manipulation or spread from carious teeth. Bacteria invade an area where turbulent blood flow passes from a high- to a low-pressure chamber, as in ventricular septal defect or mitral and aortic incompetence.

Platelets, fibrin and bacteria form friable vegetations on the damaged valve or endocardium. Aggravation of valve incompetence occurs due to destruction of endocardium, perforation of valve cusps or rupture of chordae tendinae.

Embolic incidents may occur when vegetations fragment and become detached with systemic embolism from left heart vegetations.

Pulmonary infarcts may result from vegetations originating on the pulmonary valve, ventricular septal defect or patent ductus arteriosus.

Mycotic aneurysms may develop from weakening of the muscular coats of a medium-sized artery and subsequent rupture.

The spectrum of infecting organisms include *Streptococcus viridans* from the teeth to *Streptococcus faecalis* resulting from genito-urinary instrumentation or diarrhoea.

Predisposing cardiac conditions
Mitral incompetence; aortic incompetence; bicuspid aortic valve; coarctation of aorta; pulmonary valve stenosis; small ventricular septal defect; patent ductus arteriosus.

Prosthetic valves are prone to infective endocarditis, the most common causal agents being *Streptococcus epidermitis* and fungal infection.

Tricuspid valve endocarditis is common in "main line" drug addicts. Tricuspid valve excision without valve replacement is the customary form of surgical treatment.

Clinical features
Though some patients with endocarditis show mild to moderate congestive cardiac failure, signs of systemic sepsis usually herald the presence of this serious and life-threatening condition.

Positive blood cultures are present in over 80% of cases. Antibiotic administration should be withheld until a minimum of three blood cultures have been set up.

Systemic signs
1 Splinter subungual haemorrhages
2 Clubbing of fingers
3 Splenomegaly
4 Embolic features:
   a) Osler's nodes: small tender erythematous swellings on fingers and toes
   b) Retinal emboli
   c) Focal embolic glomerulonephritis
   d) Peripheral embolisms: extremity; splenic, renal or mesenteric; cerebral; pulmonary infarction.

Cardiac manifestations
1 Murmur of the underlying endocardial or valvular predisposing lesion
2 Cardiac failure
3 Sudden development of aortic regurgitation.

Radiological chest examination and electrocardiography will help establish the nature of the cardiac lesion.

2-D echocardiography will define the cardiac defect and may demonstrate the presence of vegetations.

Treatment

Prophylactic antibiotic therapy is mandatory in patients with cardiac lesions who are to undergo dental manipulations, tonsillectomy, genito-urinary instrumentation, childbirth or gastro-intestinal operations.

Therapeutic antibiotic therapy must be used in high dosage for at least six weeks. Although a bacteriologic cure is generally possible, death from renal damage or severe valve disruption occurs frequently.

Surgical management

Indications

1 Severe congestive heart failure due to acute aortic or mitral regurgitation
2 Aortic valve replacement may be life-saving in the acute stage of infective endocarditis
3 Fresh conduction aberrations: these imply the extension of the inflammatory process from the annulus and valve leaflets into the conduction pathways. Immediate operative intervention is imperative
4 Systemic embolization: the possibility of further serious embolization may suggest the need for early cardiac surgery, unless serious cerebrovascular complications provide a contraindication to its performance
5 Prosthetic valve endocarditis is amenable to sterilization by six weeks of antibiotic treatment, but staphylococcal, gram-negative or fungal endocarditis will usually require early valve replacement.

The implantation of a prosthetic or bioprosthetic valve has to be performed carefully so that the valve can be properly positioned after all infectious material has been completely debrided.

Further Reading

Baumgartner W. A., Miller D. C., Reitz B. A. *et al.* Surgical treatment or prosthetic valve endocarditis. *Ann. Thorac. Surg.* 35: 87, 1983.

Gregoratos G., Karlwer J. S. Infective endocarditis: diagnosis and management. *Med. Clin. North Am.* 63: 1, 1979.

Lerner P. I., Weinstein L. Infective endocarditis in the antibiotic era. *New Eng. J. Med.* 274: 199, 1966.

Oakley C. M., Somerville W. Prevention of infective endocarditis. *Br. Heart J.* 45(3): 233, 1981.

Rappaport E. The changing role of surgery in the management of infective endocarditis. *Circulation* 58: 598, 1978.

Chapter 8
Aneurysms of the Thoracic Aorta

Aneurysms of the thoracic aorta may be single or multiple. They may affect the ascending aorta, the aortic arch, the descending thoracic aorta, or may be thoraco-abdominal in extent.

In addition to a traumatic cause and dissecting aneurysm which merits special consideration, the aetiologies of aortic aneurysms are:

1 *Arteriosclerotic aneurysms:* These develop at sites where atheromatous plaques have ulcerated, with ensuing weakness and thinning of the aortic wall. The aneurysms may be saccular or fusiform. The associated presence of coronary artery disease increases the operative risk to such patients (Fig. 8.1).

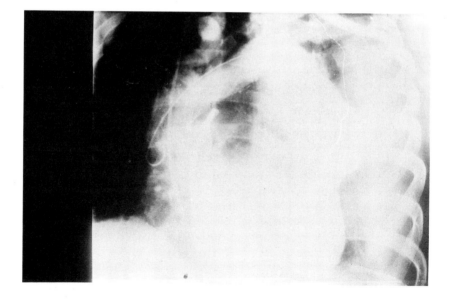

Fig. 8.1. Arteriosclerotic aneurysm of descending thoracic aorta defined arteriographically.

2 *Infective causes:* Syphilitic aneurysms are now uncommon but mycotic aneurysms due to bacterial infections of the aortic wall are likely to produce a necrotic saccular lesion in the region of the aortic annulus.

3 *Cystic medial necrosis:* This condition is most common in young males, with a special predilection for the ascending aorta. The condition may vary from aortic ectasia to a large fusiform aneurysm. Patients with Marfan's syndrome often develop a large fusiform aneurysm of the ascending aorta with involvement of the aortic annulus, causing aortic regurgitation.

4 *Takayasu aortitis:* Takayasu aortitis may give rise to aneurysms of the thoracic and thoraco-abdominal aorta.

Clinical features

Although thoracic aortic aneurysms are often asymptomatic, being discovered on a routine chest X-ray, symptoms may develop due to pressure of the aneurysm on adjacent structures. Death from rupture and exsanguination provides justification for operative intervention.
1 Pain due to pressure on chest wall or vertebrae
2 Dysphagia due to oesophageal compression
3 Respiratory symptoms due to bronchial compression
4 Hoarseness due to recurrent laryngeal nerve compression.

Radiological examination of the chest will reveal a thoracic mass, while aortography will define the vascular nature of the mass. A CT scan is a non-invasive method of confirming the diagnosis (Fig. 8.2).

Surgical treatment

Ascending aortic aneurysm

A midline sternotomy provides good access. Cardiopulmonary bypass is instituted with arterial cannulation via the aorta if feasible, or via the common femoral artery if the aneurysm extends to the arch.

After cross-clamping the aorta, the aneurysm is incised longitudinally and cardioplegia solution infused through the coronary ostia. Hypothermia reduces the myocardial temperature to 12°C. If the aortic valve is incompetent it will need to be replaced, utilizing a valved conduit. If a valved graft is used it is sutured to the aortic annulus with pledgeted 2-0 ethibond sutures. A woven preclotted dacron graft is sutured into place proximally and distally with 3-0 prolene sutures. The coronary artery ostia will be sutured circumferentially to openings made in the graft with 4-0 prolene.

The excess aneurysmal aortic tissue, after appropriate trimming, will be wrapped around the graft and secured with continuous sutures.

The operative procedure is then completed in the standard manner.

Aortic arch aneurysm
A midline sternotomy with cardiopulmonary bypass provides arterial return via the common femoral artery. Profound hypothermia with reduction of core temperature to 15° C and ice-packs

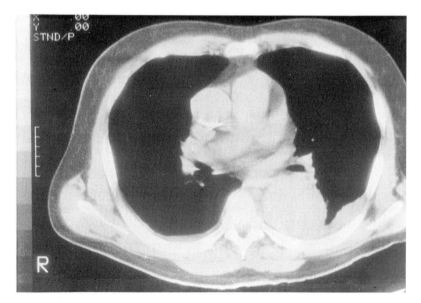

Fig. 8.2. CT scan defines extent of thoracic aortic aneurysm.

to the head will provide cerebral protection after the brachio-cephalic vessels are clamped. The descending aorta is cross-clamped and the aneurysm incised. Cardioplegia solution is infused via the coronary ostia.

Cardiopulmonary perfusion is reduced to 200 ml/min. A woven preclotted dacron conduit is anastomosed distally to the descending thoracic aorta. Bypass flow is increased to distend the anastomosis.

An oval opening at the upper end of the dacron tube allows an anastomosis between the common origin of the brachiocephalic branches and the tube, within the opened aorta.

After removing air from the graft, it is cross-clamped and the brachiocephalic clamps are removed.

The bypass flow rate is increased to 2.5 l/min and rewarming is commenced. The proximal anastomosis is completed. Needle de-airing of graft and left ventricle are completed and the patient is gradually weaned from bypass.

The wall of the aneurysm is used to buttress the graft and the operation concluded.

Aneurysm of descending aorta

A left 5th interspace thoracotomy provides adequate access. The risk of postoperative paraplegia may be avoided by use of a Gott shunt to bypass the descending aorta. The shunt is placed via prox-imal and distal purse-string sutures in the aorta. There is no need to use heparin as the shunt is coated with cationic surfactant tridodecyl-methylammonium chloride and thus is not thrombogenic.

Alternatively a femoro-femoral bypass shunt can be used but heparinization induces thoracic oozing.

Proximal and distal aortic clamps with an interposition graft replacement are not associated with a higher incidence of paraplegia than with use of the other two techniques. The graft is sutured into place proximally and distally through the opened aneurysm, after suture ligation of the intercostal artery orifices.

Thoraco-abdominal aortic aneurysm

A left abdomino-thoracic approach with division of the diaphragm permits proximal and distal clamp control of the aorta. As many intercostal arteries as can be conserved are controlled with clamp or ligature and the whole extent of the aneurysm is opened longitudinally.

After proximal anastomosis is accomplished, side openings in the graft permit early reperfusion of the coeliac, superior mesenteric, renal and inferior mesenteric arteries.

Completion of the distal anastomosis is followed by reinforcement of the fabric graft with the tailored aneurysmal tissue.

The paraplegia rate after this procedure may be as high as 25% and the operative mortality rate about 10%.

Dissecting aneurysms of the aorta

Aortic dissection is the separation of the layers of the aortic wall by haemorrhage. It occurs most commonly in hypertensive males over 40 years of age. In young people the condition occurs in association with the Marfan syndrome, in coarctation of the aorta and during pregnancy in women.

The basic pathological process is due to a weakness of the media attributable to cystic medial necrosis, which is characterized by necrosis with mucoid and cystic degeneration of the media. These changes, in turn, may be due to occlusion of local vasa vasorum.

The aorta is dissected along the weakened media by haemorrhage, producing a false lumen which communicates with the true lumen via a tear in the weakened intima. The dissection may spread along the entire length of the aorta, resulting in a "double-barrelled" aorta with occlusion of major aortic branches. The dissection may progress slowly or rapidly. The dissecting channel may perforate back into the aorta distally in about 20% of cases, with a resultant "healed" dissection which does not require surgical attention (Fig. 8.3).

Clinical features

1 Sudden onset of a severe tearing pain, usually substernal in location, is common. Depending on site of origin and extent of the dissection the pain may radiate to neck, back, abdomen and legs.

Classification

De Bakey	Shumway	Anatomic location
Type I	A	Tear just above aortic valve with dissection beyond ascending aorta or arch
Type II	A	Tear above aortic valve with dissection confined to ascending aorta or arch
Type III	B	Tear in descending aorta just below left subclavian artery

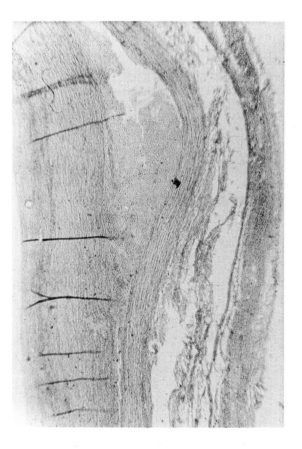

Fig. 8.3. Subintimal channel in dissecting aortic aneurysm.

2   Occlusion of aortic branches:
    a) Coronary: cause myocardial infarction
    b) Brachiocephalic arteries: changes in unilateral pulse and blood
       pressure; bizarre neurological manifestations due to impaired
       circulation to brain or spinal cord
    c) Visceral arteries: abdominal pain or renal symptoms
    d) Lower limb arteries: features of peripheral vascular disease.
3   Shock and sudden death due to rupture of the aorta into the
    pericardium, pleural cavity, abdomen or retroperitoneum.
    Failure to properly treat the condition results in death within 48
    hours in 50% of cases. Over 90% will die within the week.
4   Retrograde extension of the dissection may cause aortic
    incompetence.

Diagnosis
An index of suspicion regarding the possibility of the diagnosis
makes aortography mandatory.

Radiological examination
Widening or deformity of the aortic silhouette may be noted.
Progressive enlargement of the aortic silhouette strongly indicates
the diagnosis.
    Aortography will reveal the double aortic lumen and the extent
of the dissection. This will aid in planning the surgical approach,
whether via a midline sternotomy or a left thoracotomy.

Management
1   Sedation and analgesia
2   Reduction of high blood pressure to near normal levels by
    expeditious pharmacologic means: arfonad, nipride
3   Reduce force of left ventricular contractions: beta-blockers such
    as propranolol
4   Intravenous line; urinary catheter
5   General monitoring: ECG.

Indications for surgical treatment
1   Failure of medical treatment with progression of dissection
2   Retrograde extension with aortic incompetence

3 Compression of brachiocephalic, visceral or lower limb arteries
4 Development of pre-rupture saccular aneurysm
5 Rupture contained as false aneurysm.

Surgical techniques

Type A

Sternotomy with cardiopulmonary bypass utilizing femoral artery
for arterial inflow. Hypothermia to 28° and left ventricular venting
are instituted and the aorta is cross-clamped. The aorta is opened
transversely and cardioplegia solution is infused directly through
the coronary ostia.

If the aortic valve is incompetent, it is replaced with a biological
valve so that postoperative anticoagulation will not be necessary.
The two segments of the dissected proximal and distal parts of the
ascending aorta are sutured together and buttressed with inner
and outer rings of teflon. The two ends are then approximated
directly or via an interposed dacron tube.

Alternatively a composite valved conduit can be used with
implantation of the coronary arteries.

In very ill patients, a silicone tube can be inserted into the true
aortic lumen proximally and distally. Strong ties are applied
proximally and distally over the ascending aorta to obliterate the
dissection, squashing them down on to the splint silicone tube.

Type B

A left lateral thoracotomy provides good access to the descending
thoracic aorta. The aorta is cross-clamped above and below and
the aorta transected. The dissections are obliterated and buttressed
with teflon and aortic continuity restored by end-to-end
anastomosis or with an interposition dacron tube.

A heparinized shunt or a Gott shunt between left ventricular
apex and descending aorta can be utilized, if thought necessary, to
perfuse the lower body, viscera and spinal cord.

Aortic arch syndrome

Arteritis of the aorta and its major branches causes a broad spectrum
of clinical features with symptoms and effects dependent upon the

extent and degree of impairment of blood supply to brachiocephalic, visceral structures or lower limbs.

The aortic arch syndrome refers to the brachiocephalic component that occurs in Takayasu's disease. This condition predominantly affects young women in the Far East and Africa. The condition is also known as pulseless disease, obliterative brachiocephalic arteritis and aortic arch arteritis.

Clinical features depend upon:
1 Effects of vascular occlusion of aortic arch branches
2 Development of aortic arch aneurysms.

Aortography will define the type of architectural aberration of the vascular lesion (Fig. 8.4).

Many patients suffer from concomitant hypertension due to the pathological process also affecting the abdominal aorta with renovascular stenosis.

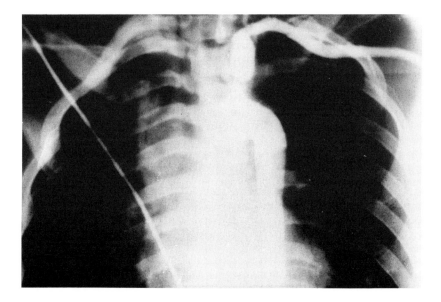

Fig. 8.4. Brachiocephalic arteritis in patient with Takayasu syndrome demonstrated arteriographically.

Treatment
Endarectomy, bypass grafts or resection with placement of inter-position grafts may be indicated.

Further Reading

Bentall H., De Bono A. A technique for complete replacement of the ascending aorta. *Thorax* 23: 338, 1968.

Crawford E. S., Crawford J. L. *Diseases of the aorta including an atlas of angiographic pathology and surgical technique.* Williams and Wilkins. Baltimore. 1984.

De Sanctio R. W., Doroghazi R. M., Buckley M. J. Aortic dissection. *N. Eng. J. Med.* 317: 1060, 1987.

Ergin M. A., Griepp R. B. Surgical management of aortic arch aneurysms. In: Cohn L. H. (ed.) *Modern techniques in surgery/cardiac thoracic surgery.* Future Publishing Co. Inc. Mt Kisco, New York. 1981.

Chapter 9
Diseases of the Pulmonary Artery

Pulmonary arteriovenous fistula

Though usually a congenital disorder, characterized by the presence of one or more cavernous haemangiomas within the lung causing arteriovenous shunting, trauma or an intrapulmonary foreign body can produce a pulmonary arteriovenous fistula.

Clinical features

Cyanosis may develop if the fistula is of significant magnitude. Dyspnoea, chest pain and haemoptysis may develop. Chronic pulmonary insufficiency with finger clubbing and polycythaemia may be present.

A continuous murmur may be audible in the pulmonary area of the fistula. Haemangiomas of the skin and mucous membranes may be present. (Osler–Weber–Rendu disease).

The arterial oxygen unsaturation due to the fistula is not improved by administration of 100% oxygen.

Radiological examination reveals a lobulated density, usually located in the lower lung field. Pulmonary angiography will establish the diagnosis.

Surgical treatment requires segmental resection or lobectomy.

Primary pulmonary hypertension

Pulmonary hypertension may be defined as an increase in pulmonary artery pressure beyond the normal (systolic: 30 mmHg: mean 8–19 mmHg).

It is usually secondary to intrinsic pulmonary or cardiac disease or to extrinsic causes of pulmonary vascular obstruction.

Primary pulmonary hypertension usually occurs in young women who present clinically with dyspnoea, syncope on effort and exertional precordial pain. As the condition progresses, cor pulmonale and right-sided heart failure develop.

Radiological examination of the chest reveals prominent pulmonary arteries and hilar vessels but diminished peripheral vascular markings.

The electrocardiogram will show features of right ventricular hypertrophy.

The aetiology of primary (idiopathic) pulmonary hypertension is not established but may be due to primary pulmonary arterial obliterative sclerosis, or pulmonary arterial thrombo-embolic disease.

Cor pulmonale

This condition represents the right ventricular hypertrophy and enlargement caused by pulmonary hypertension due to lung disease, e.g. emphysema, obstructive lung disease or cystic fibrosis. The condition does not include pulmonary hypertension due to congenital or acquired heart disease.

Irreversible pulmonary hypertension due to congenital heart disease with right to left shunting of blood is defined as the Eisenmenger complex.

Treatment of pulmonary hypertension
1 Treat cause: e.g. relief of mitral stenosis; anticoagulation for recurrent pulmonary embolism
2 Relief of airway obstruction: bronchodilators (adrenalin, aminophyllin); steroids
3 Oxygen therapy
4 Intermittent positive pressure ventilation of lungs.

Surgical management of primary pulmonary hypertension

Heart–lung transplantation is the only feasible procedure in this condition as well as in the Eisenmenger complex and selected cases of secondary pulmonary hypertension.

Criteria for heart–lung transplant
Recipients
1 End-stage parenchymal or pulmonary vascular disease
2 Age less than 45 years
3 No previous major cardiac or thoracic surgery
4 Absence of other non-reversible organ dysfunction
5 Psychosocial stability

Donor selection
1 Age under 35 years
2 Haemodynamic stability without high-dose inotropic support
3 No history of previous cardiac disease or cardiac arrest
4 No evidence of chest infection or recent chest trauma
5 No malignancy except for cerebral tumour.
There should be:
1 Approximate size and weight compatibility
2 Immunologic compatibility:
    a) Absence of donor-specific antibodies
    b) Avoid HLA–A2 mismatch.

Donor resection
The heart and lungs of the donor are removed *en bloc*. The pericardium is excised from the heart. The trachea and aorta are divided. The right atrium is opened as in a donor cardiectomy, but the left atrium is not opened and the entire unit is placed in a basin of 4°C cold saline.

Recipient transplantation
The heart and lungs of the recipient are removed separately and individually after cardiopulmonary bypass has been instituted and the anterior pericardium has been resected.

The phrenic nerves, the anterior vagus nerve on the oesophagus and the recurrent laryngeal nerve round the aortic arch with a small segment of pulmonary artery are conserved.

The donor heart and lungs are brought into the operative field and the right lung is brought beneath the caval–right atrial remnant and the right phrenic nerve to lie in the right pleural space. The left lung is placed beneath the left phrenic nerve in the left pleural space.

Reconstruction is completed in the following order using 3-0 prolene:
1 The tracheal anastomosis is performed
2 The right atrial anastomosis is completed
3 The aortic anastomosis is carried out while the patient is being rewarmed.

The aorta is de-aired, the cross-clamp removed and decannulation completed as the patient is weaned from cardio-pulmonary bypass.

Further Reading

Dines D. E., Seward J. B., Bernatz P. E. Pulmonary arterio-venous fistulas. *Mayo Clin. Proc.* 58: 176, 1983.

Griffiths B. P. Cardio-pulmonary transplantation – growing pains. *Int. J. Cardiol.* 17: 119, 1987.

Reitz B. A., Wallwork J. L., Hunt S. A. *et al.* Heart-lung transplantation: Successful therapy for patients with pulmonary vascular disease. *N. Eng. J. Med.* 306: 557, 1982.

Chapter 10
Ischaemic Heart Disease

Ischaemic heart disease is a state of insufficient coronary blood flow relative to the needs of the myocardium caused by atherosclerosis of the coronary arteries. It causes about 150 000 deaths per year in the United Kingdom and about 500 000 deaths per year in the USA. The condition is rare in Third World countries, emphasizing the relationship between nutritional and exogenous factors in causing the deposition of atheromatous material in the coronary arteries.

Atherosclerosis is a degenerative disorder leading to the deposition of plaques of lipoid material (atheroma) in the intima of arteries. Such deposition in the coronary arteries may commence in the late teens or early twenties, with involvement of multiple sites. Gradual narrowing or stenosis proceeds in the lumina of the main coronary arteries or their branches. Subintimal haemorrhage or thrombus formation may cause sudden total occlusion of such an artery.

Factors predisposing to atheroma
1 *Age*: Although faulty diet, obesity, physical inactivity, emotional stress, diabetes mellitus and family history of coronary artery disease may provide variables in age of presentation, the peak age for hospital admission with clinical features of coronary artery insufficiency is after 50 years of age. Smoking and hypertension increase the risk of ischaemic heart disease, either by accelerating atheroma deposition or by inducing coronary artery spasm.
2 *Sex*: Ischaemic heart disease shows a six-fold predominance in men over women. Females' protection may be related to sex-hormone factors. An increase in women smokers and the ingestion of contraceptive hormone pills may play a role in an increasing female incidence.
3 *Hyperlipidaemias*: Hyperlipidaemia or hyperlipoproteinaemia may be familial (Fredrickson type II) with hypercholesterolaemia or type IV with hypertriglyceridaemia causing severe atheroma in the first two decades.

Secondary hyperlipidaemia may be due to diabetes mellitus, hypothyroidism or the nephrotic syndrome.

The role of high-density lipoproteins in protecting against atheroma deposition and that of low-density lipoproteins in inducing such deposits further complicates understanding regarding relationships between high circulating levels of lipids on the one hand and atheromatous deposition on the other.

There is no irrefutable evidence to suggest that dietary or drug treatment of hyperlipidaemia reduces the risk of ischaemic heart disease. It is, however, generally asserted that saturated fatty acids (dairy products) tend to induce atheroma while unsaturated fatty acids (vegetable oils) are protective.

Clinical syndromes in ischaemic heart disease

These depend on the degree of coronary artery narrowing, the extent of collateral pathways of myocardial blood supply, or the acuity of arterial occlusion.

1 *Angina pectoris*: This clinical disorder is characterized by paroxysmal chest pain due to myocardial ischaemia, which occurs when the blood and oxygen supply to the heart is temporarily deficient to its need. Angina may be stable or unstable, nocturnal or variant (Prinzmetal).

2 *Acute coronary insufficiency*: Persistent, unremitting pain defined clinically as pre-infarction angina.

3 *Myocardial infarction*: This term indicates that necrosis of the myocardium has resulted from the decrease in blood supply. The terms coronary thrombosis or coronary occlusion are sometimes used synonymously with the term myocardial infarction. This is erroneous, confusing clinical fact with pathological cause. Cardiogenic shock may accompany a massive myocardial infarction.

4 *Cardiac failure*: This may occur because of left ventricular failure resulting from massive myocardial destruction. It may be caused by papillary muscle rupture; mitral insufficiency may follow the papillary muscle and chordae tendinae destruction; infarction of the interventricular septum with development of septal defect is a cause of severe cardiac failure.

5 *Cardiac arrhythmias* may be associated with silent or painless myocardial ischaemia.
6 *Sudden death* may be caused by ventricular tachyarrhythmias. Cardiac rupture may also be a cause of sudden death.
7 *Ventricular aneurysm*: Cardiac failure may result from the paradoxical movement of the aneurysm. Clot formation within the aneurysm or on infarcted endocardium may embolize to the peripheral arterial system. Arrhythmias are often present.

Diagnosis

Classically chest pain is described as squeezing, a sensation of precordial tightness or chest heaviness precipitated by physical effort, with cessation of pain when the exertion stops. The pain may radiate across the front of the chest, angle of jaw and neck, to the back or down both arms into the fingers.

Patients with left main coronary artery stenosis may present with effort angina or unstable angina. Persistent unremitting pain may represent pre-infarction angina.

Occasionally the patient may be pain-free and asymptomatic with a normal electrocardiograph, and a diagnosis of myocardial ischaemia is only made during an exercise tolerance test (stress test) during which severe depression of the ST segment in excess of 4 mm is registered on the electrocardiogram.

Enzyme changes (MB, CPK, SGOT, LDH): elevation of these enzyme levels indicates death of myocardial muscle and may be quantitative in its elevation.

Radio-isotope thallium-201 uptake is reduced in the area of ischaemic myocardium and may be checked as part of an exercise tolerance test.

Coronary angiography

Visualization of narrowed or occluded coronary arteries defines the extent and significance of coronary artery disease and provides criteria in patient selection for aortocoronary bypass procedures. Left ventriculography also provides information regarding its ejection capacity and whether mitral regurgitation is present.

Patient selection for aortocoronary bypass

1 Moderate to severe angina pectoris unresponsive to optimal medical therapy
2 Angiographic criteria:
  a) 50–75% stenosis of major coronary artery branches
  b) Left main coronary artery stenosis
  c) Presence of post stenotic arterial "run-off"
3 Ventricular wall haemodynamics: asynergy; ejection fraction greater than 30%; left ventricular end-diastolic pressure; presence of ventricular aneurysm; mitral valve insufficiency; presence of septal rupture
4 Ventricular arrhythmias.

Principles of medical management of myocardial ischaemia

1 Nitrates: vasodilators: reduce mechanical activity of the heart; Glyceryl trinitrate; isosorbide trinitrate may be used by sublingual, oral or transdermal routes
2 Beta-adrenergic blocking agents: reduce myocardial oxygen requirements; reverse abnormal platelet aggregations; increase haemoglobin-O_2 dissociation
3 Digitalis and diuretics
4 Anticoagulant therapy: aspirin; dipyridamole; streptokinase; tissue plasminogen activator
5 Calcium channel blockers: verapamil
6 Anti-arrhythmic agents
7 Sedation, tranquillization and oxygen therapy
8 Percutaneous transluminal angioplasty
9 Intra-aortic balloon assist device in unstable angina and cardio-genic shock

Haemodynamic monitoring in acute myocardial infarction

1 ECG monitoring for arrhythmias
2 Swan–Ganz catheter: measures cardiac dynamics, pulmonary artery end-diastolic pressure and pulmonary capillary wedge pressure
3 Arterial line: assess left ventricular function
4 Evaluate cardiac response to treatment

5 Central venous pressure line
6 Assess need for intra-aortic balloon pump support.

Percutaneous transluminal angioplasty

It is essential that a standby surgical team be available during the performance of this procedure. Immediate medical resuscitation and operative intervention is necessary if acute myocardial ischaemia is precipitated by PTA. If the sudden deterioration is due to coronary artery damage, emergency aortocoronary bypass procedure is essential.

If the patient is not in extremis, repeat angiography should be performed; if an acute occlusion is confirmed an emergency bypass procedure is indicated. Should early resolution of pain and ECG changes occur in response to medical therapy, then continued observation in the coronary care unit is justified. Any recurrence of symptoms is an indication for immediate bypass surgery.

Support by percutaneous intra-aortic balloon counterpulsation may be necessary to stabilize a patient in cardiogenic shock before the bypass operation is initiated.

During the operation it is wise to perform an arteriotomy over the thrombosed segment of the artery so that the thrombus can be removed and the dissected intima repaired before the revascularization is completed.

Historical development of myocardial revascularization

1 Interruption of pain pathways by cervical sympathectomy
2 Reduction of cardiac metabolism by induction of diminished thyroid activity
3 Extracoronary myocardial revascularization:
   a) Induction of extra-coronary vascular communications: cardio-omentopexy
   b) Intercoronary collateralization: intrapericardial talc: ligation of internal mammary artery
   c) Arteriovenous graft: narrowing of coronary sinus and aorto-coronary sinus vein graft (Beck procedure)
   d) Fresh arterial communication: tunnelling of internal mammary artery within left ventricular myocardium (Vineberg operation).

4 Direct coronary artery surgery: (Fig. 10.1)
  a) Requires cardiopulmonary bypass
  b) Reversed saphenous vein aorto-coronary graft: direct, sequential or "snake" in series
  c) Internal mammary to coronary artery anastomosis
  d) Above in combination with coronary endarterectomy
5 Combined surgery for coronary artery disease and valve replacement

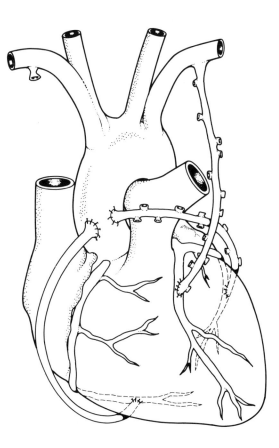

Fig. 10.1. Triple coronary bypass:
Left internal mammary artery bypass and
two saphenous vein aortocoronary bypasses.

6 Remodelling of left ventricle:
   a) Resection of akinetic area
   b) Ventricular aneurysmectomy
   c) Replacement of mitral valve
   d) Repair of ruptured septum.
7 Treatment of dysrhythmia:
   a) Resection of initiating zone
   b) Pacemaker insertion.
8 Cardiac transplantation.

Technique of aortocoronary revascularization
While the saphenous vein is being harvested, a midline sternotomy is completed and with good sternal retraction the left internal mammary artery is dissected free and is only transected after cardiopulmonary bypass is initiated; 7–0 mm prolene is used for its anastomosis to the left anterior descending artery. The right gastro-epiploic artery may be used in similar fashion. The inferior epigastric artery has been used as a free graft.

The aorta is cannulated and a two-way single atrial cannula is placed. Cardiopulmonary bypass is commenced and cooling to 25°C proceeds. The aorta is cross-clamped and cardioplegia instituted.

Adequate exposure of the left anterior descending and diagonal arteries is gained by elevating the heart on laparotomy pads.

Exposure of the marginal branches of the circumflex artery is obtained by retracting the heart anteriorly and to the right.

The right coronary artery runs in the atrioventricular groove and is often amenable to endarterectomy. Its posterior descending branch can be approached by elevating the posterior portion of the right ventricle in a cephalad direction.

After completion of the distal anastomoses the aortic cross-clamp is removed while cardiopulmonary bypass continues. Partial occlusion clamps are placed on the aorta and serial openings created for the proximal anastomoses. The patient is gradually rewarmed during this period.

Combined valve replacement and aortocoronary bypass
The left atrium or aorta is opened to expose the diseased valve which is excised. After sizing the replacement valve, the distal

coronary grafts are sutured into place. The prosthetic valve is then sutured into place and the left atrium or aorta closed. The aortic cross-clamp is removed. The heart is de-aired and while rewarming proceeds the proximal anastomoses are completed.

Left ventricular aneurysm

Left ventricular aneurysms are usually a sequel to anterior myocardial infarction resulting from occlusion of the left anterior descending artery (Fig. 10.4).

On rare occasions it is a result of trauma at a ventriculotomy site during cardiac surgery, or follows luetic, mycotic or rheumatic disease.

The aneurysmal wall of the left ventricle becomes fibrosed, with adherence of the pericardium over it. Thrombus develops within the aneurysmal sac with the capacity for peripheral embolism. The paradoxical movement of the aneurysm predisposes to the development of congestive cardiac failure.

Clinical features
After a previous myocardial infarction 15% of patients will develop an aneurysm with either:
a) Angina pectoris
b) Left ventricular failure with dyspnoea and orthopnoea
c) Systemic embolism
d) Ventricular arrhythmias.

Examination may reveal an expansile pulsation at the cardiac apex.

Electrocardiography will reveal ST segment elevation and loss of R waves persisting many months after the acute event.

Radiological examination of the chest demonstrates dilatation of the left heart border. Serial examinations may reveal progressive enlargement of the aneurysm, with calcification in its wall.

Echocardiography will define the size of the aneurysm and permit review of left ventricular global and segmental ejection fractions.

Cardiac catheterization, coronary angiography and left ventriculography will delineate the exact size and position of the aneurysm. Special note is taken regarding ejection fraction, coronary artery occlusions, whether thrombus is present and whether mitral regurgitation exists.

Surgical intervention
This is indicated if
1 A large aneurysm causes left ventricular failure
2 Embolism occurs despite adequate anticoagulation
3 Recurrent cardiac arrhythmia exists.

Aneurysmectomy
Lidocaine is administered for 48 hours before operation to prevent the development of arrhythmias. Coumarin is administered for 3 months after aneurysmectomy to prevent thrombus formation along the left ventriculotomy suture line.

A midline sternotomy provides access for cardiopulmonary bypass. The aorta is cross-clamped and cold cardioplegia solution perfused into the root of the aorta. The pericardial adhesions are freed and the heart is lifted out of the pericardial sac. The central portion of the aneurysm is incised and the intramural clot evacuated. The lateral walls of the sac are excised (Fig. 10.2).

After assurance that the mitral valve is intact, the ventricle is repaired using strips of teflon on each ventricular margin, which are incorporated within No. 1 ethibond mattress sutures. After venting the heart at the apex and removal of the cross-clamp a second suture line of continuous No. 2 prolene completes the repair.

An appropriate aortocoronary bypass procedure is carried out to revascularize the heart. The heart is defibrillated, the vent removed and the patient is weaned from cardiopulmonary bypass.

Repair of post-infarction ventricular septal defect
Two per cent of patients who suffer a transmural infarction will develop a ventricular septal defect; 50% of such patients die within the first week unless the lesion is repaired. Any unoperated survivors will develop severe congestive cardiac failure. Posterior

septal defects may occur in 30% of such patients. Involvement of the mitral valve apparatus may complicate the repair.

Utilizing cardiopulmonary bypass via a midline sternotomy the left ventricle is incised and the necrotic myocardial tissue is trimmed from both ventricles and septum until normal tissue is seen.

The septal defect is closed with a dacron patch, which is placed on the left ventricular side of the septum and on the endocardial surface of the free right ventricular wall using teflon-pledgeted prolene sutures.

The anterior infarctectomy site is then closed with a patch of low-porosity woven dacron, thereby avoiding delayed rupture of

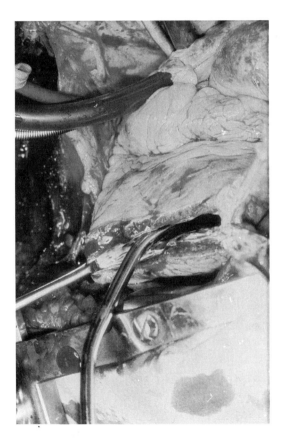

Fig. 10.2. Ventricular defect after resection of aneurysmal sac.

the ventriculotomy. The sutures along the septal margin of the left ventricle incorporate the edges of the septal patch.

The heart is de-aired, warmed and the cross-clamp on the aorta removed. The heart is defibrillated and the operation concluded.

Further Reading

Barratt-Boyes B. G., White H. D., Agnew T. M. *et al.* The results of surgical treatment of left ventricular aneurysms. *J. Thorac. Cardiovasc. Surg.* 87: 87, 1984.

Isom D. W., Spencer F. C., Glassman E. Does coronary bypass increase longevity? *J. Thorac. Cardiovasc. Surg.* 75: 28, 1978.

Loop F. D., Lytle B. W., Cosgrove D. M. *et al.* Coronary artery bypass graft surgery in the elderly, indications and outcome. *Clev. Clin. J. Med.* 55: 23, 1988.

Marks C. Historical perspectives in coronary artery surgery. *South. Med. J.* 66: 249, 1973.

Marks C., Miller A., Vidne B. Surgical treatment of left ventricular aneurysms. *Int. Surg.* 71: 69, 1986.

Ochsner J. L., Mills N. L. *Coronary artery surgery.* Lea and Febiger. Philadelphia. 1978.

Chapter 11
Diseases of the Myocardium

Idiopathic cardiomyopathy

Cardiomyopathy is a primary disorder of the myocardium. Excluded from this definition is heart disease due to congenital lesions or due to acquired rheumatic, coronary or hypertensive cardiac disorder. Also excluded are toxic causes such as alcoholism or infiltrative states such as cardiac amyloidosis or cardiac sarcoidosis.

The clinical features of this disorder may include a family history of the condition. Most frequently there is a rapid development of asymptomatic unexplained cardiomegaly, with subsequent features of congestive cardiac failure without the existence of any obvious cause.

A gallop rhythm is noted, and a diastolic murmur of aortic regurgitation or an apical systolic murmur of mitral regurgitation develops as a result of left ventricular dilatation, often disappearing with control of the congestive cardiac failure.

Episodes of tachyarrhythmia and heart block will be reflected in the electrocardiograph tracings, but sudden death is a frequent occurrence.

Types

1 *Dilated cardiomyopathy:* One or both ventricles may be affected, with failure and dilatation of the appropriate cardiac chambers. Arrhythmias and conduction defects are reflected in electrocardiographic changes, with sudden death a frequent feature. Most patients deteriorate progressively despite treatment of cardiac failure, use of beta-blockers, vasodilator and anti-arrhythmic agents. Anticoagulants may be necessary to prevent thrombo-embolic episodes.

2 *Hypertrophic cardiomyopathy:* Thickening of the left ventricle may obliterate its cavity, with marked thickening and immobility of the septum. Obstruction of the left ventricular outflow tract is often defined as hypertrophic obstructive cardiomyopathy with

75

significant pressure gradients. The condition is often familial in
incidence, presenting as an autosomal dominant characteristic.

Clinical features include angina, syncope, dyspnoea and
rhythm disorders.

Echocardiography defines the thickened immobile septum,
the small left ventricular cavity and the systolic anterior motion
of the mitral valve.

Administration of beta-blockers may be helpful but surgical
relief may require:

a) Resection of focally hypertrophied muscle

b) Mitral valve replacement for associated mitral insufficiency

c) Cardiac transplantation.

3 *Restrictive cardiomyopathy:* This condition may mimic the clinical
features of constrictive pericarditis due to the restriction of
cardiac filling. The marked cardiomegaly is associated with great
hypertrophy and dilatation of all the cardiac chambers, with
mural thrombi present in 25% of cases. The coronary arteries
are normal without any areas of stenosis, thereby excluding an
ischaemic aetiology. The specific sub-types are:

a) Endomyocardial fibrosis: this condition is common in West
and Central Africa. The dominant feature is fibrosis of the
endocardium with involvement of the papillary muscles and
chordae of the mitral and tricuspid valves

b) Fibroelastosis of infancy with thickening of endocardium
and clinical features of congestive heart failure.

Surgical treatment

The only prospect of survival for young patients with the various
forms of cardiomyopathy depends upon the successful performance
of a heart transplant.

Primary endocardial fibroelastosis

The primary form of endocardial fibroelastosis causes congestive
heart failure within the first year of life, with death by 2 years of
age.

During the period of gestation, the endocardium of the left
atrium and left ventricle becomes very thick. Intrauterine infection,

bacterial or viral, anoxia and other non-specific hereditary traits may provide aetiological factors, as there is a significant familial incidence.

Primary endocardial fibroelastosis must be differentiated from the secondary endocardial fibrotic thickening that occurs in coarctation of the aorta, aortic stenosis and other types of congenital heart disease.

Clinical features

The infant appears normal in the early months of life. The left ventricle then begins to hypertrophy until cardiac failure occurs, with tachycardia, tachypnoea, dyspnoea and hepatomegaly.

Cardiomegaly distorts the left side of the heart and pulmonary hypertension develops rapidly.

No murmurs are audible unless mitral insufficiency develops.

Radiological examination confirms the gross cardiomegaly.

Electrocardiography reveals left ventricular hypertrophy and strain.

2-D echocardiography confirms the hypertrophied left ventricle with its restricted mobility. There will be an absence of intracardiac shunts or other congenital anomalies.

Cardiac catheterization will demonstrate normal to slightly elevated right ventricular pressure, but a markedly elevated left ventricular end-diastolic pressure.

Angiocardiography will confirm the restricted motion of the left ventricle, with its minimal ejection fraction.

Surgical treatment

1 Endocardial resection has limited value
2 Heart transplantation and, in the presence of pulmonary vascular resistance above 8 Wood units, heart–lung transplantation provide the only hope for cure.

Kawasaki's disease

This multisystem disorder of unknown aetiology affects children under 5 years of age. It is characterized by acute systemic manifestations which are followed by cardiovascular sequelae such as coronary and peripheral artery aneurysms, coronary artery stenoses and mitral valve insufficiency, that are amenable to surgical amelioration.

Heart transplantation
Indications
1 Cardiomyopathy   53%
2 Myocardial ischaemia   35%
3 Congenital heart disease   8%
4 Other   4%

Recipient selection
Irremediable terminal cardiac disease with less than 10% likelihood of surviving for 6 months.
1 Age: 60 years or younger
2 Normal function or reversible dysfunction of liver and kidneys
3 Absence of infection
4 Absence of recent pulmonary infarction
5 Absence of insulin-dependent diabetes mellitus
6 Absence of pulmonary vascular resistance greater than 8 Wood units.

Donor matching
1 ABO blood type compatibility
2 Absence of donor-specific lymphocyte cytotoxicity
3 Appropriate size match: weight and body surface area
4 HLA–A2 compatibility.

A recipient post-transplant immunosuppressive regimen will require a fine balance between the desired benefit of the drugs and their potential adverse effects.

Prednisone, azathioprine (imuran) and cyclosporine represent the pharmacological mainstay of immunosuppressive therapy in heart transplantation. Monitoring of rejection episodes requires endomyocardial biopsy and histological grading techniques, although M-mode echocardiography, electrocardiographic changes and cardiac radionuclide scanning may provide non-invasive methods of indicating rejection.

Radio-immune assay of serum levels of cyclosporine during treatment must be performed permitting a level of 200–400 ng/ml, with subsequent adjustment to less than 200 ng/ml if no rejection episodes develop.

Technique of heart transplantation

Donor cardiectomy

After administration of intravenous heparin (3 mg/kg) the heart is exposed via a midline sternotomy. The aorta, pulmonary artery and venae cavae are dissected out. The aorta is cross-clamped and cold cardioplegia solution infused into the aortic root to achieve cardiac arrest and rapid cooling of the heart.

The venae cavae are ligated and divided. The left atrium is incised for decompression of the left ventricle and the incision is continued circumferentially at the level of the pulmonary veins. The aorta and pulmonary artery are transected and the heart is immersed in cold saline. It is then placed in two concentric bags, each containing iced saline and the entire collection is placed in an ice-container for transportation.

Before its transplantation the left atrium is opened by a connecting incision between the pulmonary vein orifices and trimmed. This provides a single left atrial chamber for anastomosis.

The ligated superior vena cava remnant is secured with a transfixion suture, while the inferior vena cava orifice is left open.

The aorta and pulmonary artery are dissected apart for their anastomosis to the recipient's arteries.

Orthotopic heart transplantation

The recipient's diseased heart is exposed via a midline sternotomy. The aorta is cannulated and two venous cannulae are placed. Caval tapes are tightened to provide total cardiopulmonary bypass and the patient is cooled to 25°C. The aorta is cross-clamped and the recipient's heart is excised by incisions in the atria just posterior to the atrioventricular groove. The aorta and pulmonary artery are transected distal to their valves and the heart is removed.

The donor heart now replaces the removed diseased heart. The left atrium of the donor is anastomosed to the recipient's left atrium starting at the atrial appendage and continuing circumferentially, using a long double-armed 3-0 prolene suture, until the atrial septal union has been completed (Fig. 11.1).

A catheter is inserted through the left atrial appendage into the left ventricle, with an infusion of cold saline for myocardial preservation.

The donor right atrium is opened upwards from the open inferior vena cava remnant in oblique fashion, so as to avoid the sinoatrial node at the superior vena cava–atrial junction.

The right atrial anastomosis is completed with full-thickness sutures through the septal area of the left atrial anastomosis.

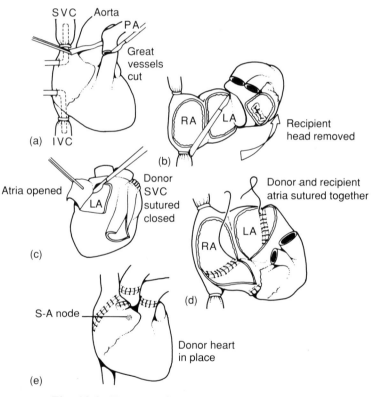

Fig. 11.1. Donor and recipient cardiac chambers sutured in course of orthotopic heart transplantation.

The aortic and pulmonary anastomoses are then carried out with 4-0 continuous prolene sutures while rewarming is initiated. The aortic root is de-aired, the heart is defibrillated and the patient gradually weaned from cardiopulmonary bypass.

Heterotopic heart transplantation
The patient's own heart is left *in situ*, continuing its functional activity if transplant rejection necessitates removal of the donor heart.

The recipient is placed on cardiopulmonary bypass in the standard manner.

The left atrium is incised for its entire length and the donor left atrium is anastomosed to it in a side-to-side manner.

The donor ascending aorta is anastomosed end-to-side to the recipient aorta; the donor superior vena cava is anastomosed to the side of the recipient's superior vena cava.

The donor pulmonary artery is anastomosed to the recipient's main pulmonary artery either directly or using an interposed dacron graft.

The danger of a low flow state in the transplanted heart and the risk of thrombo-embolism requires permanent postoperative anticoagulation.

Cardiac lesions in the carcinoid syndrome
Hyperserotoninaemia due to the excessive production of 5-hydroxytryptamine is the result of functional carcinoid tumours of the small intestine which have metastasized to the liver. The diagnosis of the carcinoid syndrome is supported by finding elevated urinary levels of 5-hydroxy-indole acetic acid (5-HIAA).

The clinical features of skin flushing, diarrhoea and broncho-spasm may be complicated by cardiac involvement, with tricuspid insufficiency or pulmonary stenosis leading to right heart failure and death.

The cardiac changes are predominantly those of fibrosis of the valves of the right heart, leading to pulmonary stenosis and tricuspid stenosis, or regurgitation with sclerosis and partial fusion of the cusps. As the lung has a high monoamine oxidase content which inactivates serotonin, it is rare for the mitral and aortic valves to be affected.

Serotonin production by primary malignant bronchial carcinoma may, however, exert similar pathological lesions on the valves of the left heart.

Surgical relief of the valvular disorder can now be successfully accomplished by valve replacement.

Further Reading

Barnard C. N. A human cardiac transplant. *South African Med. J.* 41: 1271, 1969.

Barnard C. N., Barnard M. S., Cooper D. K. *et al.* The present status of heterotopic cardiac transplantation. *J. Thorac. Cardiovasc. Surg.* 81: 433, 1981.

Bierman F. Z., Gersony W. M. Kawasaki disease: Clinical perspectives. *J. Pediatr.* 111: 789, 1987.

Dye C. L., Genovese P. D., Daly W. J., Behnke R. H. Primary myocardial disease: II, Haemodynamic alterations. *Ann. Int. Med.* 58: 442, 1963.

Fay W. P., Taliercio C. P., Ilstrup D. M. *et al.* Natural history of cardiomyopathy in the elderly. *J. Am. Coll. Cardiol.* 16(4): 821, 1990.

Goodwin J. F., Gordon H., Hollman A., Bishop M. B. Clinical aspects of cardiomyopathy. *Br. Med. J.* 1: 69, 1961.

Kelly J., Andersen D. H. Congenital endocardial fibroelastosis: Clinical and pathologic investigation of those cases without associated cardiac malformations including report of two familial instances. *Paediatrics* 18: 539, 1956.

Lower R. R., Sofer R. C., Shumerksy N. E. Homoviral transplantation of the heart. *J. Thorac. Cardiovasc. Surg.* 41: 196, 1961.

Marks C. *Carcinoid tumors.* G. K. Hall & Co. Boston. 1979.

Oyer P. E., Stinson E. B., Jamieson S. W. *et al.* One year experience with cyclosporine A in clinical heart transplantation. *Heart Transplant* 1: 285, 1982.

Chapter 12
Acquired Chronic Valvular Disease

The sinister nature of rheumatic fever is predominantly due to the structural changes which complicate acute rheumatic valvulitis. Neither the concomitant myocarditis nor the pericarditis of the acute episode leaves any significant residual dysfunction.

Acquired valvular disease is almost always rheumatic in origin. Rarely, syphilitic aortitis and atherosclerosis are aetiological factors.

In half of all cases there is no history of an acute rheumatic episode, implying that the process is usually subclinical.

The left heart is affected much more frequently than the right:
1 Mitral valve in 80% of cases
2 Aortic valve in 50% of cases
3 Tricuspid valve in 10% of cases
4 Pulmonary valve: never.

Haemodynamics
The deformed valve interferes with function in two ways:
1 *Stenosis*: Fusion and thickening of valve cusps reduces the diameter of the open valve orifice with obstruction to the prograde flow of blood. The heart chamber behind the stenotic valve undergoes compensatory hypertrophy, but progressive restriction of flow occurs and by the time the stenotic valve is reduced to 25% or less of normal, decompensation and cardiac failure become overt.
2 *Incompetence*: Contraction, distortion and fusion of valve cusps prevents their complete apposition, allowing retrograde leakage when the valve is closed resulting in valve incompetence or regurgitation.

Valve incompetence may result from dilatation of the fibrous ring to which the leaflets are attached, as in syphilitic aortitis and acute rheumatic carditis.

Ventricular dilatation can stretch the atrioventricular valves causing functional tricuspid or mitral incompetence without the presence of organic valvular disease.

Rupture or perforation of a valve cusp by ulcerative

destruction in bacterial endocarditis can also cause valvular incompetence.

Rheumatic valvular deformity may cause stenosis, incompetence or a combination of the two.

Mitral valve disease

Mitral stenosis

The normal mitral valve area measures 4–6 cm^2. Mitral stenosis results from fusion and fibrous thickening of the valve leaflets and their chordae tendinae. If the valve remains flexible without shortening of the chordae there may not be any associated valve incompetence, but in most cases some degree of mitral insufficiency coexists. Tight stenosis of an extreme degree is represented by a funnel-shaped type of stenosis with a very small aperture 0.5–1.5 cm^2 (Fig. 12.1).

The narrowed mitral valve orifice obstructs blood flow through it, with a rise in left atrial pressure which is duly transmitted to the pulmonary veins and capillaries with transudation of fluid into the pulmonic interstitial tissues. There is a coincidental elevation of pulmonary artery pressure which results in right ventricular strain and hypertrophy.

Clinical features

A slight degree of mitral stenosis is compatible with a long symptom-free life. As the valve orifice falls below 1.8 cm mild symptoms begin to develop with dyspnoea on strenuous activity that did not cause symptoms before. As the orifice falls below 1.5 cm, shortness of breath is precipitated by ordinary activity such as walking rapidly, and slight orthopnoea.

With a valve orifice under 1 cm the capacity for effort is markedly reduced, with severe orthopnoea and episodes of paroxysmal nocturnal dyspnoea.

Haemoptysis may occur because of pulmonary congestion or infarction. Cough is a frequent symptom. Hoarseness and dysphagia may be due to pressure by the enlarged left atrium.

Complications

1 *Atrial fibrillation*: This complication, the result of left atrial stress, is present in 50% of cases. Its onset may precipitate an episode of pulmonary oedema or congestive cardiac failure. Less often atrial tachycardia or flutter may complicate mitral stenosis.

2 *Pulmonary infections*: Recurrent bronchitis and broncho-pulmonary infections frequently occur.

3 *Pulmonary arterial hypertension*: Vasoconstrictive pulmonary hypertension leads to right ventricular failure and secondary tricuspid insufficiency. Thrombo-obstructive pulmonary artery disease will lead to episodes of pulmonary infarction and

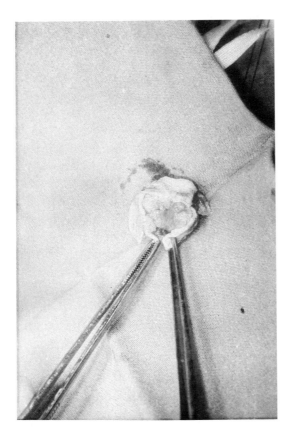

Fig. 12.1. Resected stenosed mitral valve.

haemoptysis. Irreversible pulmonary hypertension may develop in long-standing cases.

4 *Left atrial thrombosis* results from the stagnation of blood in the left atrium. Systemic arterial embolism, especially to the brain, results from detachment of a portion of thrombus.

5 *Congestive heart failure* may be secondary to pulmonary hypertension or to the onset of atrial fibrillation. Pregnancy may precipitate its onset, mitral stenosis being more common in females. The New York heart classification grades the severity of symptoms from I (mild) to IV with severe congestive heart failure.

6 *Bacterial endocarditis*: This complication is more likely to affect the incompetent mitral valve than the purely stenotic one.

7 *Compressive effects of large left atrium*: Dysphagia from oesophageal compression, hoarseness due to paralysis of the left recurrent laryngeal nerve, pulmonary collapse and infection from compression of the left main bronchus.

Clinical examination

A mitral diastolic murmur that varies from mid-diastolic to the entire diastolic period in relation to mild and severe stenosis is diagnostic.

Electrocardiography may reflect a P mitrale in severe stenosis if sinus rhythm is present. Atrial fibrillation may be noted.

Radiological examination of the chest may show the enlarged left atrium, Kerley's lines or septal lines at the lung bases, as well as pulmonary venous congestion. Valve calcification may be seen (Fig. 12.2).

Echocardiography will define the nature of the valvular disorder, the presence or absence of vegetations and the left atrial dimension. A left atrial thrombus, if present, will be noted. The degree of leaflet mobility is assessed. The aortic and tricuspid valves are viewed for stenosis and regurgitation.

Cardiac catheterization is indicated only rarely; resting left atrial pressure and pulmonary pressure can be monitored with a Swan–Ganz catheter and is an essential investigation to assess pulmonary vascular resistance in advanced cases.

Surgical treatment of mitral stenosis
Closed mitral commissurotomy
This procedure is indicated in cases of pure mitral stenosis uncomplicated by associated valvular incompetence. The procedure is contraindicated if the leaflets are calcified, or in patients with atrial fibrillation or leaflet vegetations.

The procedure is performed through either a left anterolateral or posterolateral 5th interspace thoracotomy. After opening the pericardium, the left atrial appendage is delivered and a vascular clamp placed at its base. A purse-string suture is brought through

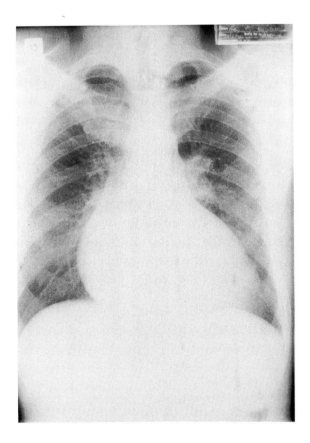

Fig. 12.2. Left atrial enlargement, demonstrated radiologically, due to recurrent mitral stenosis 8 years after closed mitral valvotomy.

a snare. The appendage is incised and the clamp is released, washing out any atrial thrombus.

The finger is inserted through the purse-string suture and the valve is explored for presence or absence of regurgitation. The anterolateral and posteromedial commissures are then gently opened by finger fracture without tearing the left atrium.

If a good commissurotomy cannot be done with finger fracture, then a purse-string suture at the apex and a left ventriculotomy permits the passage of a Tubbs dilator, which is guided to the atrial finger for dilatation of the stenotic valve.

After dilatation is complete, the atrial finger is withdrawn, the appendage re-clamped and the purse-string suture is tied and reinforced with an oversewing suture. The clamp is removed and the operation concluded.

Cardiopulmonary bypass facility should be available in case mitral regurgitation develops, so that immediate valve replacement or reconstruction can be done.

Open mitral commissurotomy

A midline sternotomy permits cardiopulmonary bypass to be instituted. Cooling to 30°C proceeds; the aorta is cross-clamped and cardioplegia infused into the aortic root. The left atrium is opened and proper retraction exposes the mitral valve, which is inspected. Elevation of the valve leaflets exposes the chordae tendinae. The commissural fusion is relieved and the chordae tendinae freed. If necessary the Tubbs dilator can enlarge the mitral orifice and valve competence is then tested by injecting saline under pressure into the left ventricle and checking for regurgitation.

With a satisfactory commissurotomy completed, the left atrium is closed, the heart de-aired and decannulated after warming, and the operation terminated.

Mitral valve replacement

After opening the left atrium, the mitral valve is excised with the chordae tendinae and tips of the papillary muscles resected sufficiently to avoid interference with the valve function. During the excision and valve replacement it must be remembered that the circumflex artery in the posterior atrioventricular groove is vulnerable to a deep suture and that the proximity of the A-V node to the anterior leaflet and posterior commissure may expose it to damage and heart block.

After excision of the valve, sizers will indicate the diameter of the prosthesis, with the directive to use a valve that is a little too small than one a little too large.

2-0 pledgeted dacron sutures are used to sew the prosthetic valve into place, using either continuous or interrupted sutures. Commencing at the anterior commissure the suturing proceeds clockwise and is completed when the valve is finally in place with the sutures secured. After removal of the valve-holder, a small catheter is inserted through the valve into the left ventricle (Fig. 12.3).

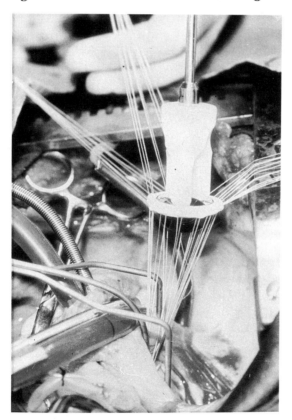

Fig. 12.3. Prosthetic valve being sutured into mitral position after excision of the diseased valve.

As the heart is allowed to fill with blood, air is removed from the heart, the left atrium is closed and the catheter is removed.

The heart is rewarmed, the aortic cross-clamp removed, de-airing completed and after decannulation the procedure is concluded with pacer wires attached and exteriorized.

Mitral regurgitation

The mitral incompetence or insufficiency that causes to and fro movement of blood across the mitral valve may be due to:
1   Rheumatic valvulitis
2   Subacute bacterial endocarditis
3   Trauma: blunt or penetrating cardiac trauma, surgical trauma to cusps, chordae or papillary muscles at closed mitral valvotomy
4   Myocardial infarction with rupture of papillary muscle or chordae.

Haemodynamics

During ventricular systole there is regurgitation of blood into the left atrium, thereby reducing the prograde flow into the aorta. During ventricular diastole the left atrial flow includes the pulmonary venous inflow volume plus the previously regurgitated amount, distending the left ventricle and causing left ventricular dilatation and hypertrophy.

A pansystolic apical murmur with a soft first sound and a third heart sound is audible.

A P mitrale is seen electrocardiographically unless atrial fibrillation is present.

Enlargement of the left atrium and left ventricle are seen on X-ray of the chest, while echocardiography will determine the state of the valve and heart chambers (Fig. 12.4).

Angiocardiography will provide visualization of the contrast material opacifying the left atrium as it regurgitates during left ventricular contraction.

Surgical management

Although mitral valve replacement may be necessary if the valve cusps are rigid and calcified, reconstruction of the mitral valve should be performed whenever possible. It is advantageous for the patient to retain the natural valve mechanism and not to require post-replacement anticoagulation.

Reconstructive techniques for mitral regurgitation

The procedures, carried out via a midline sternotomy and cardiopulmonary bypass, has a low operative mortality (3%) with a 10-year survival of 90%. A third of the patients may require further valve surgery after 10 years. The prolonged period of palliation has special merit in children, allowing time for them to grow before valve replacement might become necessary.

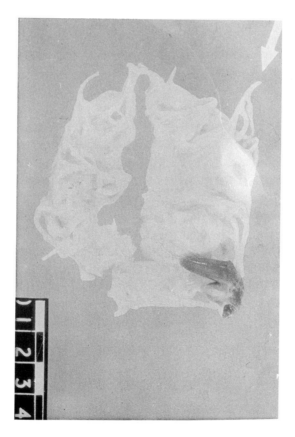

Fig. 12.4. Resected incompetent mitral valve.

1 *Perforation of a leaflet*: If the rest of the valve mechanism is normal or reparable, the perforation may be treated by sewing in a patch of pericardium.
2 *Annuloplasty*: As the valve leaflets thicken and scar, the valve leaflets cannot come together during ventricular systole, causing regurgitation. Dilatation of the annulus can be remedied by an annuloplasty that will reduce the diameter of the annulus by plication utilizing an annuloplasty ring.

A Carpentier–Edwards rigid ring systematically plicates the posterior leaflet while maintaining the area of the anterior leaflet.

The flexible Duran or Pugia–Massala ring provides a simple technique for narrowing the mitral annulus. Plication of a redundant scallop of the posterior annulus may be necessary. A quadrilateral resection of the posterior leaflet may be appropriate if rupture of the posterior chordae causes the regurgitation. The leaflet tissue is then resutured and the repair reinforced with an annuloplasty ring.
3 *Repair of ruptured chordae*
   a) Anterior leaflet: rupture of anterior leaflet chordae can be repaired by transfer of chordae from the posterior leaflet with its suture to the free edge of the anterior leaflet. The unsupported segment of the posterior leaflet is then resected.
   b) Shortening the elongated chordae: whether attached to the anterior or posterior leaflets, the elongated slack chordae can be shortened by creating an incised trench in its papillary muscle. The chordal tendon is then tautened and drawn into the trench and sutured into position, shortening it according to the depth of the trench.
   c) Ruptured or elongated papillary muscle: rupture or excessive elongation of a papillary muscle may be caused by a myocardial ischaemic event resulting in excessive leaflet motion. The papillary muscle may be repaired or reimplanted in the free wall of the left ventricle. The elongated papillary muscle may be shortened by plication or by implantation in a trench created in the left ventricular wall.
   d) If there is associated mitral stenosis, the valve may be salvaged by debridement and curettage of calcium from the anterior

leaflet, with division of the commissures of the chordae tendinae and papillary muscles.

Increasing experience indicates that mitral valve repair has a great prospect of success in rheumatic valvular disorder as well as in mitral insufficiency secondary to ischaemic heart disease.

Further Reading

Braunwald E. Valvular heart disease. In: Braunwald E. (ed.) *Heart disease: A textbook of cardiovascular medicine.* 2nd ed. W. B. Saunders Co. Philadelphia. 1984.

Carpentier A. Cardiac valve surgery – the French correction. *J. Thorac. Cardiovasc. Surg.* 86: 383, 1983.

Kirsh M. M., Sloan H. Technique of mitral valve replacement. *Ann. Thorac. Surg.* 30: 490, 1980.

Souttar H. J. Surgical treatment of mitral stenosis. *Br. Med. J.* 2: 603, 1925.

Yellin E. L., Yoran C., Frater R. W. M. Physiology of mitral valve flow. In: Duran C., Angell W. W., Johnson A. D., Ovry J. H. (eds.) *Recent progress in mitral valve disease.* Butterworth. London. 1984.

Chapter 13
Acquired Aortic Valve Disease

Aortic stenosis

Aortic valve calcific stenosis in the adult invariably complicates a bicuspid valve of congenital origin. It results from fusion of the valve leaflets at their commissures followed by scarring, thickening and distortion of the valve cusps. The affected valve becomes rigid and calcified. Aortic regurgitation may accompany the stenosis (Fig. 13.1). Rheumatic aortic stenosis may develop as a result of thickening and fusion of the cusps.

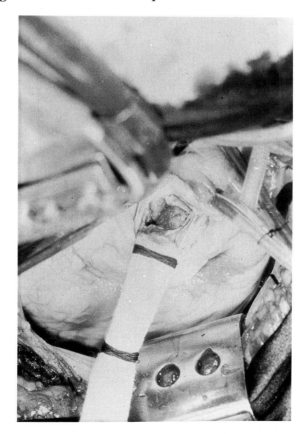

Fig. 13.1. Operative view of diseased aortic valve prior to excision.

Aortic stenosis causes specific haemodynamic changes:

1 Systolic gradient across the valve: The pressure, during systole, is greater in the left ventricle than in the aorta. When the valve area, calculated utilizing the Gorlin formula, falls to less than 1 cm, the gradient becomes higher than 50 mmHg. At such gradient levels, surgical intervention is generally advisable.

2 Left ventricular hypertrophy is confirmed by electrocardiography, which demonstrates left axis deviation and possible patterns of left ventricular strain, reflected in ST wave depression and T wave inversion.

Clinical features

There is usually absence of any circulatory disturbance until the valve area is reduced by about 50%. The earliest symptoms are related to decreased coronary and cerebral blood flow and to reduced systemic output.

1 *Angina pectoris*: The chest pain, brought on by exertion and relieved by rest, is attributable to inadequate coronary blood flow.

2 *Syncope*: Light-headedness or syncope, due to insufficient cardiac output and cerebral blood flow, occurs after exertion and may be the only manifestation of aortic stenosis.

3 Fatigue or dyspnoea after light exertion occurs because of reduced systemic output. Progressive left ventricular failure leads to congestive cardiac failure.

4 Sudden death is not uncommon and may be due to arrhythmias e.g. ventricular fibrillation, myocardial infarction or cerebral ischaemia.

5 Effects of bacterial endocarditis may intervene.

Auscultation of the chest reveals a loud systolic ejection murmur which stops before the second sound is heard. It is transmitted into the neck. There may be a diastolic murmur of associated aortic regurgitation.

In advanced aortic stenosis the peripheral pulse is of low amplitude. It rises and falls slowly (pulsus parvus et tardus).

Radiological examination of the chest may show significant left ventricular enlargement. There may be post-stenotic aortic dilatation, with calcification of the stenosed valve.

Echocardiography will reveal diminished cusp mobility and valve calcification as well as its effects on the cardiac chambers.

Cardiac catheterization and angiography will define the severity of the stenosis. It will delineate associated regurgitation, coronary artery disease and concomitant mitral valve disease.

The aortic orifice area can be calculated from Gorlin's formula:

$$\text{Area} = \frac{\text{Mean systolic flow in ml/s}}{44.5 \text{ mean systolic gradient between l.v. and aorta}}$$

Surgical management

1 Percutaneous transaortic balloon aortoplasty may be indicated in some very poor-risk cases.
2 Commissurotomy is occasionally indicated in patients with a trileaflet valve and absence of calcification. Calcium debridement alone may sometimes restore normal leaflet mobility.
3 Aortic valve replacement is generally indicated.

Aortic valve replacement

A midline sternotomy and cardiopulmonary bypass with hypothermia and cardioplegic arrest is carried out. The aortic valve is exposed through an oblique aortotomy well above the coronary artery ostia. Cardioplegia may need to be initiated via the coronary ostia if associated regurgitation is present. A vent is placed in the left ventricle via a left atriotomy and the aortic valve is visualized.

The aortic leaflets are excised with three commissural traction sutures in place. The valve orifice is sized and the replacement valve selected. Interrupted pledgeted mattress sutures of 2-0 braided polyester are passed through the three aortic annular areas, alternating different coloured sutures. These are then passed through the sewing ring of the prosthetic valve which is then placed and the sutures tied (Fig. 13.2).

The aortotomy is closed with 3-0 prolene sutures while the patient is being rewarmed. The aortic cross-clamp is removed, the aorta and left ventricle are de-aired. The patient is weaned from bypass, decannulated and the operation concluded.

Enlargement of aortic annulus diameter

If the annulus is unduly small, with a diameter less than 19 mm prohibiting the insertion of an adequately sized valve prosthesis, then enlargement of the annulus by 2–3 mm is possible.

1 *Nick's operation*: After the aortic leaflets have been removed an incision is made into the non-coronary sinus of Valsalva, thereby dividing the annulus. The incision can be extended to the upper trigone of the mitral leaflet. A wedge-shaped dacron patch is sutured in place as a posterior annular patch. This enlarges the circumference of the annulus permitting the implantation of a full-sized prosthesis. The aortotomy is then closed by sewing the remaining part of the patch into place in the aortic wall.

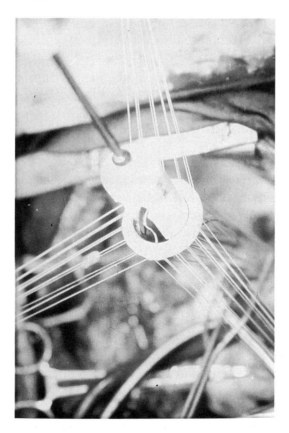

Fig. 13.2. Prosthetic valve being sutured into aortic position.

2 *Konno operation*: If enlargement of the annulus is needed for
   patients with significant subannular fibromuscular obstruction
   then, after excision of the valve leaflets, a vertical incision in the
   aortic annulus is extended into the right coronary cusp well to
   the left of the right coronary orifice and is extended transversely
   into the right ventricle 1 cm below the pulmonary valve orifice.

   A high incision is made in the interventricular septum, away
   from the conduction pathway, joining the aortotomy and thereby
   opening up the entire left ventricular outflow tract.

   A diamond-shaped dacron patch is tailored for suturing into
   the septotomy, across the annulus to the aorta, thereby enlarging
   the annulus significantly by suturing each end of the divided
   annulus to the patch.

   The valve prosthesis is sutured circumferentially to the natural
   annulus and the enlarged bridge of dacron patch with continuous
   3-0 dacron suture.

   The rest of the patch is used to close the anterior aortotomy
   with 4-0 prolene sutures.

   A pericardial patch is then fashioned for suture at the base of
   the dacron and folded back to close the right ventriculotomy.

Left ventricular apico-aortic conduit

In conditions such as tunnel stenosis of the left ventricle and other
obstructive lesions of the left ventricular outflow tract that preclude
prograde flow, the interposition of a conduit between the left
ventricular apex and the thoracic or abdominal aorta provides a
ready solution to the problem of outflow obstruction to the left
ventricle.

Standard cardiopulmonary bypass is instituted if a midline
sternotomy is required to assess the aortic lesion.

A conduit between the cardiac apex and the descending aorta
can be readily accomplished via a left 6th interspace thoracotomy
utilizing a left atrium to femoral artery bypass.

The apex of the left ventricle is exposed, a ventriculotomy with
removal of a plug of myocardium establishes a site for insertion of
a flanged cannula, which is sutured into place.

A valved conduit is sutured to the intracardiac cannula and
then anastomosed to the selected aortic site.

Aortic regurgitation

If the aortic valve becomes shrunken, fibrotic and distorted aortic incompetence will result. During diastole, the left ventricle will fill by backflow through the aortic valve in addition to the blood received from the left atrium. In order for this increased diastolic volume to be accommodated, the left ventricle undergoes dilatation and hypertrophy.

Aetiology

1 Rheumatic valvulitis: most common cause
2 Bacterial endocarditis: the features of sepsis, a positive blood culture of streptococcus or staphylococcus is an indication for immediate aortic valve replacement after completion of antibiotic therapy. This complication may affect the natural valves or a prosthetic valve
3 Syphilitic aortitis
4 Dissecting aneurysm
5 Aneurysm of ascending aorta e.g. Marfan's syndrome
6 Trauma: blunt, penetrating or iatrogenic.

Clinical features

Patients may remain asymptomatic for many years without deterioration, with only an audible aortic diastolic murmur, as the heart undergoes its compensatory changes. In the penultimate stage of the disease, severe congestive failure develops.

Physical examination demonstrates the classic features of a widened pulse pressure, low diastolic pressure and heightened aortic and systemic arterial pulsations.

Expressions of these haemodynamic changes are reflected in the "collapsing pulse", "waterhammer pulse", Corrigan's sign, De Musset's sign; "pistol-shot" femoral artery sounds; Durosiez's sign.

Radiological examination of the chest may reveal cardiomegaly, dilatation of the aorta and occasionally calcification in the aortic valve area.

Electrocardiography reflects left ventricular hypertrophy with tall T waves in V5 and V6.

Echocardiography demonstrates a large, dilated, vigorous left ventricular cavity with aortic incompetence. When cardiac decompensation develops the left ventricular contractions become poor and weak.

Cardiac catheterization and aortography will define the amount of regurgitation of aortic contrast material into the left ventricle (Fig. 13.3).

Treatment
An asymptomatic patient with an aortic diastolic murmur due to aortic regurgitation without cardiomegaly may be observed at 6-monthly intervals. If heart enlargement develops or clinical deterioration is observed, then aortic valve replacement should be recommended.

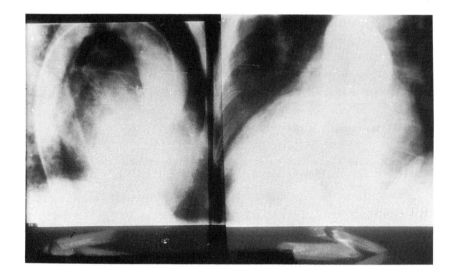

Fig. 13.3. Aortic valve incompetence with regurgitation of contrast material into left ventricle.

Further Reading

Frank S., Johnson A., Ross J. Jr. Natural history of valvular aortic stenosis. *Am. Heart J.* 35: 41, 1975.

Henry W. L., Bonow R. O., Rosing D. R., Epstein S. E. Observations on the optimum time for operative intervention for aortic regurgitation: I, Serial echocardiographic evaluation of asymptomatic patients. *Circulation* 61: 484, 1980.

Konno S., Imay Y., Nakagrume M. *et al.* A new method for prosthetic valve replacement in congenital aortic stenosis associated with hypoplasia of the aortic valve ring. *Bull. Heart Inst. (Japan)* 15: 1, 1974.

Scott W. C., Miller D. C., Haverich A. *et al.* Determinants of operative mortality for patients undergoing aortic valve replacement. Discriminant analysis of 1,479 operations. *J. Thorac. Cardiovasc. Surg.* 89: 400, 1985.

Chapter 14
Acquired Tricuspid Valve Disease

Tricuspid stenosis
Almost all cases of acquired tricuspid stenosis are rheumatic in origin, with concurrent mitral valve disease; 5% of patients undergoing mitral valve surgery will have varying degrees of tricuspid stenosis. Other causes of acquired tricuspid stenosis include the carcinoid syndrome and disseminated lupus (Libman–Sacks disease).

Clinical features
Right-sided heart failure results in liver congestion, ascites and peripheral oedema. The raised jugular venous pressure, the enlarged tender liver, ascites and dependent oedema are associated with a diastolic murmur audible in the tricuspid area.

Chest X-ray may demonstrate right atrial enlargement but features of mitral valve disease will usually be superimposed.

The electrocardiogram will show P pulmonale as a result of right atrial enlargement.

Echocardiography reveals a tricuspid valve altered to the same shape as in mitral stenosis, and an enlarged right atrium.

Cardiac catheterization will reveal a valvular gradient if simultaneous right atrial and right ventricular pressures are taken.

Treatment
As tricuspid valvotomy produces tricuspid regurgitation, valve replacement is the only effective procedure. In the placement of sutures in the annulus to fix the prosthesis, avoidance of the A-V node is necessary.

Tricuspid regurgitation
1 *Organic*: Rheumatic fibrosis and deformity of the valve with shortening and fusion of the chordae leads to valvular incompetence. Mitral disease is usually also present.
2 *Functional regurgitation*: Right ventricular failure and dilatation, usually aggravated by atrial fibrillation, widens the tricuspid annulus and renders the tricuspid valve incompetent.

3 *Bacterial endocarditis* in "mainline" drug addicts has become a
   potent cause of tricuspid regurgitation.

Haemodynamics

During ventricular systole, blood regurgitates through the
incompetent tricuspid valve into the right atrium. During right
ventricular diastole the combination of this blood volume plus
that arriving from the great veins provides an increased volume
load on the right atrium and right ventricle, causing both chambers
to dilate and undergo hypertrophy.

Clinical features

A rise in right atrial pressure leads to jugular vein distension,
pulsatile hepatomegaly with ascites and signs of congestive failure.

A pansystolic murmur at the lower end of the sternum becomes
louder with inspiration.

Chest X-ray and electrocardiography reveal cardiomegaly due
to enlargement of the right atrium and ventricle with right ventricular hypertrophy.

Echocardiography reveals a large right ventricle.

Cardiac catheterization and angiography will demonstrate
systolic regurgitation of right ventricular contrast material into the
right atrium.

Surgical treatment

Tricuspid regurgitation often accompanies mitral valve disease. A
right atriotomy will permit visualization of the tricuspid valve and
a decision is made to reconstruct or replace it. A left atriotomy then
permits the definitive mitral valve procedure. Restoration of tricuspid competence is then accomplished by two optional methods.

1 *The De Vega technique*: Plication of the tricuspid annulus is
   achieved by using a double-armed 'O' prolene suture which
   transfixes the ring at the antero-septal commissure and continues
   circumferentially to the level of the coronary sinus orifice. The
   suture is tied over a pledget at each end so as to reduce the
   annular diameter by one third.

2 *A Pugia–Massala ring* is fixed to the annulus by a continuous 'O'
   prolene suture. The contained suture within the M-P ring is

then tightened to reduce the tricuspid annular area to the desired diameter and secured.

If there is leaflet fibrosis or fixity, the leaflets should be resected and valve replacement carried out.

Further Reading

Arbula A., Asfan I. Tricuspid valvectomy without prosthetic replacement: Ten years of clinical experience. *J. Thorac. Cardiovasc. Surg.* 82: 684, 1984.

Rivera R., Duran E., Ajuria M. Carpentier's flexible ring versus De Vega annuloplasty. *J. Thorac. Cardiovasc. Surg.* 89: 196, 1985.

Chapter 15
Valve Prostheses

No artificial valve is as perfect as the healthy functional natural valve. Each prosthetic valve has potential advantages and disadvantages which need to be considered in making a final choice for placement at a specific site in an individual patient.

The perfect artificial valve should subscribe to certain specifications:

1 *Durability*: The prosthetic valve should last for the probable life span of the patient. At the present time an unmounted homograft in the aortic position is the most durable. Mechanical valves of the monostrut, low profile or convex–concave type endure for up to 10 years while biological or tissue valves tend to disintegrate or calcify within 6 years.

2 *Haemodynamic efficiency*: The valves should be sensitive to low gradients for easy flow at the atrioventricular sites. The blood flow area should be adequate with minimal turbulence.

3 *Thrombogenicity*: Mechanical valves are highly thrombogenic because of blood turbulence at its interface with the device. Thrombosis may occlude the valve and embolism to brain or elsewhere may have catastrophic consequences. The St. Jude's valve appears to be the least thrombogenic of the mechanical valves. The life-long administration of oral anticoagulants such as warfarin is mandatory after insertion of mechanical valves. Regular control of the coagulation state by the plasma thromboplastin time is also necessary. Tissue valves and unmounted homograft are less thrombogenic and do not require anticoagulant therapy.

4 *Tissue compatibility*: There is no problem with rejection or incompatibility with any of the three categories of valve prostheses.

5 *Ease of insertion*: Mechanical and biological valves require the same technical approach in their surgical implantation. The implantation of homografts requires specialized experience and skill.

6 *Cost*: There is little difference in the cost of the different varieties of prostheses.
7 *Endocarditis*: This is a rare complication and is less likely to occur in tissue valves.
8 *Silence*: The click of the mechanical valve does not appear to worry patients. Tissue and homograft valves are totally silent.

Types of current valve prostheses

Mechanical valves
1 Ball and cage: Starr–Edwards; Smeloff–Cutter. A cloth-covered cage with a hollow metal ball of Stellite 21. These have the disadvantage of cage protrusion with possible irritation of the ventricular septum and obstruction of the left ventricular outflow tract.
2 Pivoting disc: Bjork–Shiley; Medtronic–Hall; Lillihei–Kaster. The disc valves have a low profile with a short excursion of the disc. There is less haemolysis and less likelihood of outflow tract obstruction (Fig. 15.1).
3 Hinged disc: St Jude's: functionally efficient with lowest index of thrombogenicity amongst the mechanical valves.

Biological or tissue valves
Calf pericardium; dura mater or pig valves are mounted on a titanium frame covered in dacron. The tissues are fixed in glutaraldehyde and sterility is maintained by formaldehyde. The deleterious effects of sterilization include disintegration or calcification of the valve within 5–7 years. Improvement in durability has accompanied glutaraldehyde-fixation sterilization methods.

Ionescu–Shiley valve: calf pericardium; Hancock or Carpentier–Edwards valves: pig valves. The efficacy of St Jude's bio implant has enjoyed recent emphasis (Fig. 15.2).

Homograft valves
Antibiotic sterilized homograft valves are obtained from fresh cadavers and stored at 4°C. These valves can be inserted into the aortic position by free-hand suture without the use of a stent.

Complications associated with prosthetic valves
Early complications:
1 Prosthetic dislodgement due to suture disruption
2 Embolism: thrombus, calcific debris, air
3 Distortion of adjacent valve by too large a prosthesis
4 Myocardial perforation during insertion of prosthesis with serious haemorrhage
5 Malfunction: especially in ball-valve type prosthesis with protrusion of papillary muscle, chordae or teflon margin of ring into the device

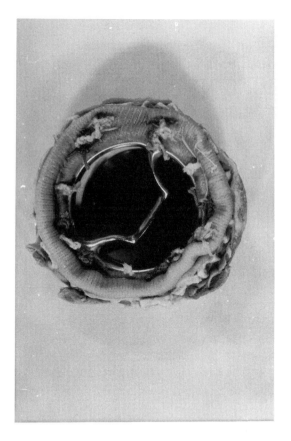

Fig. 15.1. Bjork–Shiley mitral disc valve prosthesis.

6 Injury to adjacent structures: trauma to conducting pathway; suture through coronary arteries

7 Stenosis of valve orifice by thrombus.

Late complications:

1 Thromboembolism

2 Bacterial endocarditis

3 Paravalvular leak

4 Haemolytic anaemia if prosthesis becomes regurgitant in aortic position

5 Loss of ball in ball-valves; loss of valve

6 Strut fracture of pivoting disc valve.

Further Reading

Arom K., Nicoloff D. M., Kersten T. E. *et al.* St. Jude medical prosthesis: Valve related deaths and complications. *Ann. Thorac. Surg.* 43:491, 1987.

Barratt-Boyes B. G. Long-term follow-up of aortic valvar grafts. *Br. Heart J.* 33 (suppl.): 60, 1971.

SPECIFICATIONS

The St. Jude Medical* BioImplant™ heart valve is available in tissue anulus sizes 23 mm to 32 mm.

Model	Position	Tissue Anulus Diameter (mm)	Orifice Diameter (mm)	Profile Height (mm)
A-783-23	Aortic	23	20.0	9.5
A-783-24	Aortic	24	21.0	10.0
A-783-25	Aortic	25	22.0	10.5
A-801-27	Aortic	27	24.5	10.8
A-801-28	Aortic	28	25.0	11.5
M-801-28	Mitral	28	25.0	11.5
M-801-30	Mitral	30	27.0	13.0
M-801-32	Mitral	32	29.0	14.0

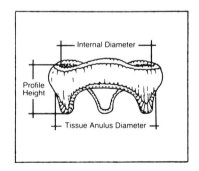

Fig. 15.2. St Jude's bioimplant.

Barratt-Boyes B. G., Roche A. H. G. A review of aortic valve homografts over a six and a half year period. *Ann. Surg.* 170: 483, 1969.

Bjork V. O., Henze A. Ten year experience with the Bjork–Shiley tilting disc valve. *J. Thorac. Cardiovasc. Surg.* 78: 331, 1979.

Ross D. N. Replacement of aortic and mitral valve with a pulmonary autograft. *Lancet* 2: 956, 1967.

Chapter 16
Tumours of the Heart

Primary cardiac tumours may be classified as pericardial, myo-cardial or intracavitary. These tumours may be benign or malignant, and malignant tumours may be primary or metastatic.

Metastatic tumours

These are 25 times as common as primary heart tumours. Metastatic tumours of the heart are predominantly carcinomas, the most common primary sites being lung and breast. The oesophagus, thyroid, thymus and genito-urinary tract may provide the sites of the primary cancer. Invasion of the heart may be by direct extension, by retrograde lymphatic spread or by haematogenous dissemination.

Mesenchymal sarcomas, lymphomas and lymphosarcoma may involve the heart. Malignant melanomas may develop cardiac metastases.

Primary malignant tumours

Sarcomas account for 20% of all primary cardiac neoplasms occurring in adults without predilection for males or females. The right atrium is most often affected, with origin from endocardium or pericardium. These highly malignant tumours rapidly infiltrate all layers of the heart and adjacent mediastinal structures. Systemic metastases are present in the majority of cases, with early spread to lungs and mediastinal lymph nodes.

Fibrosarcoma, angiosarcoma, myxosarcoma and rhabdomyo-sarcoma as well as Kaposi sarcoma have all been described. A rare tumour is the primary osteogenic sarcoma of the heart (Fig. 16.1).

These patients rapidly develop congestive cardiac failure, cardiomegaly, haemopericardium, arrhythmia and sudden death. Intracavitary extension may occlude the tricuspid valve and the orifices of the venae cavae.

Benign tumours

75% of primary tumours are benign, with myxomas comprising over 50% of the lesions. Rhabdomyoma is the most common tumour found in children and represents 20% of all benign tumours. Rarely fibroma, lipoma, haemangioma, teratoma or mesothelioma may be found.

Limbl's excrescence is a rare papillary tumour of the aortic valve and adjacent endocardium in adults, or of the tricuspid valves in children, and represents a variant myxoma.

Myxoma

Representing half of all primary heart tumours, the myxoma consists of a polypoid mass of gelatinous material most frequently located in the left atrium. It may, less often, be found in the right atrium or either ventricle.

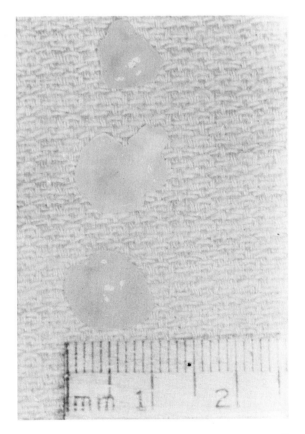

Fig. 16.1. Resected three distinct primary osteogenic sarcomas of heart chambers.

Though benign, the tumour may recur locally if not completely removed. The tumour is usually attached by a pedicle to the fossa ovalis, atrial appendage or pulmonary vein (Fig. 16.2).

Atrial myxomas may occur at all ages but are most commonly found in middle-aged females.

A familial form (Carney's syndrome) of atrial myxoma has been described in sets of siblings or parent offspring. Familial tumours are more common in young males. The tumours may be multicentric and may be associated with eyelid myxomas, Cushing's syndrome and adrenocortical nodular dysplasia. In females labial lentiginosis and bilateral myxoid mammary fibroadenomata have been described.

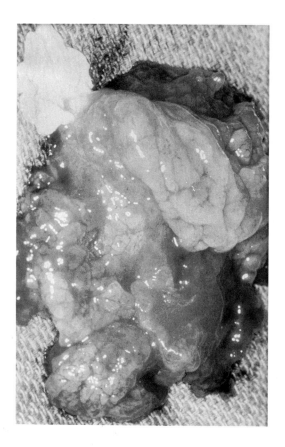

Fig. 16.2. Resected left atrial myxoma with pedicle of normal endocardium.

Clinical features

Primary heart tumours usually produce symptoms that, although protean in pattern, indicate a need and justification for surgical excision.

1 *Mass effect*: An intracavitary tumour may obstruct blood flow through the cardiac chamber or may interfere in "ball-valve" fashion with the normal opening and closure of the adjacent valves. Left atrial myxomas will affect the mitral valve, with features of intermittent mitral stenosis and development of pulmonary hypertension. Dyspnoea, syncope, angina, peripheral oedema and ascites are the predominant features, with a possible murmur suggestive of valvular stenosis or incompetence.

    Neoplastic infiltration of the myocardium by a malignant mural tumour will cause chest pain and myocardial dysfunction with congestive failure. Involvement of conduction pathways will cause arrhythmias, heart block and Stokes–Adams episodes.

2 *Embolization*: Systemic emboli from fragmentation of left atrial myxomas most commonly involve the central nervous system, which may provide the earliest symptoms. Right heart tumours rarely cause pulmonary embolism.

3 *Constitutional symptoms*: Fever, malaise, weight loss, elevated sedimentation rate, polymyositis and hepatic dysfunction are frequently associated with left atrial myxomas. These effects are probably produced by interleukins released by the tumour.

    Haemolytic anaemia and thrombocytopaenia may represent the result of blood cell destruction by a mobile intracavitary tumour.

    The occasional occurrence of polycythaemia with right atrial tumours may be a response to hypoxia induced by tricuspid valve obstruction, elevation of right atrial pressure, stretching of the foramen ovale and a resultant right to left shunt.

Diagnosis

Radiological chest examination may demonstrate non-specific cardiac enlargement. Rarely tumour calcification may be seen in a right atrial myxoma or in osteogenic sarcoma.

    Electrocardiography is rarely helpful though arrhythmia or cardiac chamber enlargement may be noted.

Cardiac catheterization and angiography, though diagnostic, is neither necessary nor desirable as it may precipitate tumour embolization. The presence of an intracavitary filling defect does not differentiate between tumour and other intracardiac masses such as thrombus, abscess, vegetation or aneurysm.

2-D echocardiography will demonstrate the pedunculated or sessile nature of the tumour and may reveal the mobility of the left atrial myxoma as it moves in and out of the mitral orifice. Cardiac contractions can be gauged with provision of enough information to permit surgical intervention. (Fig. 16.3).

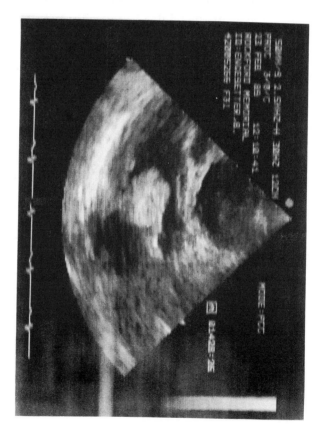

Fig. 16.3. Atrial tumour defined at echocardiography.

Surgical treatment

A midline sternotomy provides access for total cardiopulmonary bypass, hypothermia and cardioplegic arrest.

The left atrium is opened posterior to the interatrial groove and the tumour visualized. A counter-incision is then made in the right atrium along the sulcus terminalis, with careful preservation of the sinus node.

The fossa ovalis in the interatrial septum is incised circumferentially and the tumour and its endocardial base delivered through the left atrial incision.

The interatrial defect is then closed with a continuous 4-0 prolene suture. The left atrial incision is closed after placement of a trans-mitral vent. The right atrial incision is closed and venous tourniquets are removed, allowing the right heart to fill.

The aortic cross-clamp is removed, the heart is de-aired and warmed and after completion of venting, the vent is removed.

The patient is gradually weaned from bypass and the operative procedure concluded in standard manner.

Further Reading

Carney J. A. Differences between non-familial and familial cardiac myxoma. *Am. J. Surg. Path.* 9: 53, 1985.

Chitwood W. R. Cardiac neoplasms: Current diagnosis, pathology and therapy. *J. Cardiac Surg.* 3: 119, 1988.

Dein J. R., Frist W. H., Stinson E. B. *et al.* Primary cardiac neoplasm: Early and late results of surgical treatment in 42 patients. *J. Thorac. Cardiovasc. Surg.* 93: 502, 1987.

Klima T., Milam J. D., Bossart M. I., Cooley D. A. Rare primary sarcomas of the heart. *Arch. Path. Lab. Med.* 110: 1155, 1986.

Larriev A. J., Jamieson W. R. E., Tyers G. F. O. *et al.* Primary cardiac tumors: Experience with 25 cases. *J. Thorac. Cardiovasc. Surg.* 83: 339, 1982.

PART III
CONGENITAL DEFECTS OF THE HEART

Chapter 17
General Diagnostic Features

The presence of congenital heart disease may be suspected because of certain symptoms and clinical features such as dyspnoea, failure to grow and thrive and recurrent episodes of pulmonary infection.

Clubbing of fingers and toes or the presence of a precordial thrill and murmur may be noted on clinical examination.

Aetiological factors in congenital heart disease

In the past, cardiac malformations were attributed either to developmental errors or to fetal endocarditis. By 1941, it became generally known that maternal rubella during the first trimester of pregnancy often caused cardiac malformations such as patent ductus arteriosus and ventricular septal defects.

High altitude: Maternal hypoxia among people living in high-altitude regions may influence the higher incidence of patent ductus arteriosus.

Genetic factors: Patent ductus arteriosus, atrial and ventricular septal defects as well as other congenital cardiac malformations may be transmitted through several generations, or may be noted in siblings.

Associated congenital defects

The genetic basis of the cardiac anomalies may be reinforced by the presence of congenital heart disease in known hereditary disorders.

1 *Marfan's syndrome (arachnodactyly)*: The long slender limbs, poor muscle tone, laxity of ligaments, hypermobility of joints and scoliosis are associated with a high arched palate, ocular abnormalities with subluxation of the lens, myopia, microcornea, strabismus and nystagmus.

    The cardiovascular component in this dominant genetic condition is present in 25% of patients. Aortic root ectasia, ascending aortic aneurysm and dissecting aneurysm are frequently present. Coarctation of the aorta, patent ductus arteriosus and atrial septal defects may occur.

119

2 *Ellis van Creveld syndrome*: Chondroectodermal dysplasia, polydactylism and ventricular or atrial septal defects are found.
3 *Trisomy 21 (mongolism)* is accompanied by congenital heart disease in 30% of cases.
4 *Gargoylism with valvular abnormalities*: Endocardial fibroelastosis both have a genetic determinant.
5 *Turner's syndrome* i.e. Chromatin-negative XXY females with gonadal dysgenesis may suffer from coarctation of the aorta and other congenital heart anomalies.
6 *Noonan syndrome*: Pulmonary valve dysplasia with hypertelorism and skeletal abnormalities.

The relationship between virology, genetics and environment in causing aberrations of cardiac development seems clear.

In children, as in adults, cardiac surgery falls under two headings:
1 *Open heart surgery*: An open heart procedure is one in which extracorporeal circulation or cardiopulmonary bypass is employed to maintain the functional capacity of the cardiac and respiratory systems during the operation.
2 *Closed heart procedures*: These are operations in which extracorporeal circulation is not used.

Diagnosis in suspected congenital heart disease

Clinical manifestations
1 *Poor feeding*: There is an inability or lack of desire in the infant or child to take its feed, readily noticed by nurse or mother. Failure to thrive or gain weight is a byproduct of poor feeding, and is common in cyanotic congenital heart disease e.g. Tetralogy of Fallot.

Tiredness and dyspnoea may be the earliest symptom of congenital heart disease. Children may prefer a squatting posture to relieve the dyspnoea.
2 *Rapid respiratory rate*: As a sign of early heart failure, the sleeping respiratory rate of an infant may increase to over 60 per minute. Associated difficulty in breathing represents dyspnoea and in the acyanotic infant suggests a left to right shunt with early heart failure.

3 *Recurrent respiratory infections* are common in congenital cardiac malformations with congested lungs. Exercise tolerance is usually diminished.

4 *Cyanosis*: This denotes a right to left intracardiac shunt as in Tetralogy of Fallot, tricuspid stenosis, transposition of the great arteries, truncus arteriosus and anomalous pulmonary venous drainage.

   If reversal of blood flow develops with flow from pulmonary artery to aorta in patent ductus arteriosus, cyanosis is predominant in the lower limbs.

5 *Miscellaneous signs*
   a) Clubbing of fingers and toes develops after the development of cyanosis in the cyanotic form of congenital heart disease. Polycythaemia develops in response to the arterial oxygen unsaturation.
   b) Pulse characteristics: strong pulses in upper limbs and weak in lower limbs is characteristic of coarctation of the aorta. Collapsing pulse is associated with patent ductus arteriosus, weak pulses are associated with pulmonary stenosis.
   c) Prominence of the left precordium develops from long-standing right ventricular hypertrophy pressing against a soft and pliable chest wall.

6 *Heart murmurs*: This is a significant physical sign, when present it is often associated with a palpable thrill. It may be found in an asymptomatic child or may be associated with signs of heart failure or cyanosis.

   Murmurs in neonates are usually systolic. In patent ductus arteriosus, the machinery murmur only becomes characteristic in older children. Murmurs heard in the first 24–48 hours of life are usually due to an obstructive lesion, e.g. aortic stenosis; those developing later generally suggest septal defects.

   The quality of the second heart sound is important. A split second sound indicates the closure of normal aortic and pulmonary valves.

   A single unsplit second sound is heard in aortic or pulmonary atresia, persistent truncus arteriosus and severe forms of Fallot's Tetralogy.

Neonatal heart failure

The commonest congenital cardiac lesions causing heart failure are:

1 *Within 2 weeks of age*
   a) Hypoplastic left heart
   b) Obstructive left heart lesions: coarctation of aorta or aortic stenosis.

2 *After 2 weeks of age*
Usually occurs with large left to right shunts manifesting as the natural pulmonary vascular resistance lessens:
   a) Atrial septal defect, ventricular septal defect or patent ductus arteriosus
   b) Truncus arteriosus
   c) Double outlet right ventricle
   d) Severe endocardial cushion defect.

3 *Probability relative to age*
   a) At birth: hypoplastic left ventricle
   b) 1–7 days:
      i) Patent ductus arteriosus
      ii) Transposition of great arteries
      iii) Total anomalous pulmonary venous drainage.
   c) 7–14 days:
      i) Aortic stenosis
      ii) Pulmonary stenosis
      iii) Coarctation of the aorta.
   d) 14–30 days:
      i) Ventricular septal defect
      ii) Atrioventricular septal defect.

Neonatal cyanosis
Inspection of the lips, tongue, tip of nose, conjunctiva, oral mucous membranes and nail-beds of fingers and toes will provide evidence of existent cyanosis.

The radiological presence of cardiomegaly in association with cyanosis is diagnostic of a congenital heart defect.

Persistent cyanosis despite breathing 100% oxygen strongly indicates congenital heart disease. The disappearance of cyanosis on pure oxygen implies:

1 It is pulmonary in origin and may be attributable to a persistent fetal circulation
2 Total anomalous pulmonary venous connection (the only congenital cardiac condition responsive to oxygen)
3 Central nervous depression or lung disease.

Specific lesions causing cyanosis in the neonate
1 *Transposition of the great arteries*: This is the commonest cause of neonatal congenital cyanotic heart disease. Persisting patency of the ductus arteriosus permits communication between the pulmonary and systemic circulations. Intermittent patency of the ductus may cause intermittent cyanotic episodes responsive to prostacyclin therapy.
2 *Pulmonary atresia*: With or without a ventricular septal defect
3 *Total anomalous pulmonary venous return* (responsive to oxygen therapy)
4 *Tricuspid atresia*.

Congenital heart disease in children
These may be categorized as cyanotic or acyanotic forms.

Acyanotic congenital heart disease
• Ventricular septal defect
• Atrial septal defect
• Patent ductus arteriosus
• Aortic stenosis
• Coarctation of the aorta
• Left heart lesions: mitral stenosis, cor triatrium
• Aortic arch anomalies
• Pulmonary stenosis
• Ebstein's anomaly.

Cyanotic congenital heart disease
- Tetralogy of Fallot
- Transposition of the great arteries
- Truncus arteriosus
- Anomalous pulmonary venous drainage
- Tricuspid atresia
- Pulmonary atresia.

Radiological examination
Specific details may aid in diagnosis:
1 *Size and contour*: General cardiomegaly or chamber enlargement may be characteristic for several congenital heart defects:
   a) Boot-shaped heart or *coeur en sabot* of Fallot's Tetralogy.
   b) The "figure-of-eight" or "cottage loaf" shape of total anomalous pulmonary venous drainage.
   c) The narrow vascular waist of transposition of the great arteries
   d) The wide vascular waist of truncus arteriosus.
2 *Pulmonary blood flow*: There is decreased blood flow to the lungs, with diminished vascularity of the lung fields in tricuspid atresia and in pulmonary stenosis and atresia, and in Fallot's Tetralogy.
      Increased blood flow in the pulmonary arteries leads to increased vascularity of the lung fields. With great increase in the volume of pulmonary blood flow, the pulmonary arteries become large and pulsate with a recognizable "hilar dance" at fluoroscopy. This state will occur with shunts of blood from left to right heart or through a patent ductus arteriosus.

Electrocardiography
The normal neonate demonstrates right ventricular dominance in distinction to the evolution of left ventricular dominance in the normal adult. Evaluation of an abnormal electrocardiogram in association with the pattern of pulmonary blood flow and the presence or absence of cyanosis permits anatomic inferences regarding the clinical probability of the types of congenital heart disorder, e.g. a cyanotic infant with pulmonary oligaemia with electrocardiographic evidence of left ventricular hypertrophy will have tricuspid atresia and/or hypoplastic right ventricle. Contrarily, right ventricular hypertrophy would be indicative of Fallot's Tetralogy.

In acyanotic cases left to right shunts (e.g. atrial septal defects) or obstruction to the right ventricular outflow tract will demonstrate right ventricular hypertrophy. Left ventricular hypertrophy will be associated with uncomplicated patent ductus arteriosus, aortic stenosis, coarctation of the aorta.

High or peaked P waves express the presence of atrial enlargement.

In dextrocardia the leads reveal a mirror-image of the normal pattern.

Anomalous origin of the left coronary artery from the pulmonary artery will demonstrate deep wide Q waves, raised ST segments and inverted T waves characteristic of myocardial ischaemia.

Disturbance of conduction may be revealed with non-specific prolongation of PR interval; partial or complete right bundle branch block is commonly associated with ostium primum forms of atrial septal defect.

Echocardiography

Current 2-dimensional echocardiography can provide accurate diagnosis of the anatomic disorders in congenital heart disease without need, in many cases, of invasive investigational procedures.

Imaging: Ultrasound is high-frequency sound above the audible range of 50–20 000 Hz but frequencies of 1.9–7.5 MHz are used for examining the heart. There is better penetration at the lower and higher resolution at the upper end of this range.

A piezoelectric crystal is made to vibrate by the passage of an electric current. This generates a pulse of ultrasound that travels through the body at 1540 miles/s. Most of the transmitted sound energy is absorbed or scattered, but some is reflected at the interface between tissues of differing acoustic impedance, e.g. pericardium and myocardium.

The returned reflected pulses are detected by a receiving crystal and recorded as a spot on a display screen. The position of the spot is determined by the time difference between the transmission and the return of the pulse.

To form a typical two-dimensional sector, scan pulses are transmitted along about 120 scan lines over a 90 arc 30 times per second (Fig. 17.1).

An M mode image is constructed by transmitting and recording at only one of these scan lines and displaying the returning echoes as a graph of depth against time (Fig. 17.2).

Doppler ultrasonography

The shift in frequency between transmitted and reflected ultrasound defines velocity. As red blood cells flow towards the transducer they shorten the ultrasound wavelength; as they move away they lengthen it.

The audiosignal reflects the shift in frequency and guides the transducer to obtain the best visual display.

Computerized analysis of the returning ultrasound signal plots velocity against time. The density of a point on the display screen is proportional to the number of red cells moving at that velocity.

The degree of valvular stenosis can be measured: normal laminar flow across the mitral valve has a narrow range of blood velocity. With the development of stenosis, peak velocity rises, the rate of decay of peak velocity falls and as flow becomes turbulent a greater range of velocities develops.

Techniques

1 *Continuous wave*: two crystals for transmitting and receiving. Though sensitive to high maximal velocities, there is poor localization of abnormal flow areas.
2 *Pulsed Doppler*: A single crystal transmits pulsed ultrasound and receives echoes after timed delay. Localization within an echocardiographic image is possible at specific depths of tissue.
3 *Colour flow Doppler*: This system calculates mean blood velocity and direction of flow at multiple points down each scan line of an image sector. The velocity data are then superimposed on to the echocardiographic image with colour coding which helps the visual detection of abnormal flows. This reduces the need for cardiac catheterization.

Flow towards the transducer is displayed as red, flow away from the transducer as blue.

Aliasing represents changes in velocities with changes of colour from red to blue or vice versa at points of abnormal flow.

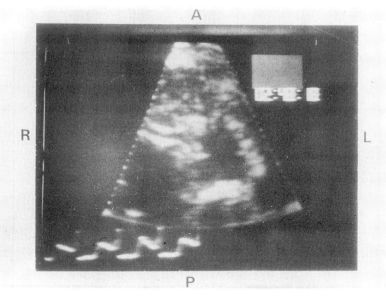

Fig. 17.1. 2-D echocardiogram defines left atrial membrane.

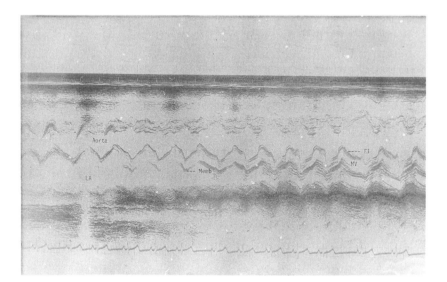

Fig. 17.2. M-mode image of left atrial membrane.

Some systems substitute green for red and blue at such sites of high variance, which highlights turbulent flow.

The ultrasound examination

Views: 1 Parasternal
        2 Apical
        3 Subcostal
        4 Endoscopic transoesophageal.

Sector and colour flow scans utilize parasternal and apical views to provide rapid review of morphological and haemodynamic abnormalities.

The subcostal view provides good imaging of the interatrial septum.

M mode recordings through the aortic valve, mitral valve and left ventricle are taken before use of the continuous wave Doppler.

The apical view is used to record mitral and aortic flow. The aortic valve can be viewed via the right intercostal spaces; the pulmonary valve via left parasternal position and the aorta from the suprasternal notch.

Endoscopic transoesophageal transducers can image the entire thoracic aorta, the atria, interatrial septum and proximal left coronary artery.

Vegetations and thrombi are better defined by transthoracic echocardiography, as are aortic dissections.

Intraoperative or postoperative monitoring of intracardiac mitral reconstructive procedures is possible by this technique.

The injection of microbubbles into peripheral veins may delineate areas of coronary artery stenosis and their haemodynamic significance.

Cardiac catheterization

First performed on himself by Werner Forssman in 1929, with passage of a catheter from the left forearm into the right atrium. In 1941 Cournand and Ranges defined the procedure as a diagnostic tool in heart disease and after the introduction of extracorporeal circulation by Gibbon in 1953, its important role in correct preoperative diagnosis was emphasized. Although echocardiography has supplanted the routine use of cardiac catheterization, it remains an important investigative technique.

Indications
1 To provide anatomic data in complex heart defects.
2 To provide physiological data:
  a) Pulmonary and systemic blood flows and their ratios
  b) Total pulmonary artery resistance
  c) Pulmonary arteriolar resistance
  d) Ratio of pulmonary and systemic resistance
  e) Calculation of left to right and right to left shunts.
3 To assess location and severity of obstructive lesions of pulmonary, aortic, mitral or tricuspid stenosis or shunts, utilizing indicator dilution curves.
4 Evaluation of ventricular function:
  a) Left end-diastolic pressure (EDP)
  b) Rate of change of pressures (dp/dt)
  c) End-systolic volume
  d) Diastolic volume
  e) Ejection fraction.
5 PO_2 saturation in various cardiac chambers using oximeter.

Angiocardiography
This will delineate the nature and site of arterial stenoses or the nature of abnormal intracardiac shunts. Selective radio-opaque contrast material e.g. caesium iodide is injected through the catheter, viewed through an image intensifier and recorded angiographically. Mitral or aortic regurgitation can be similarly recorded.

Technique
Under local anaesthesia in adults or general anaesthesia in children, a catheter is inserted through an antecubital vein and passed into right atrium, right ventricle and pulmonary arteries. Pressures are recorded in each chamber and blood samples withdrawn for oxygen saturation studies. A Swan–Ganz balloon catheter wedged into the pulmonary arterioles will record equivalent left atrial pressures. Trans-arterial catheters can be similarly passed into the left ventricle.

Results

1 Visualization of catheter: diagnostic inference may be drawn from the abnormal site of a catheter as it passes through a septal defect, patent ductus arteriosus or anomalous pulmonary vein.
2 Oxygen saturation: the sudden increase in oxygen saturation in:
   a) Right atrium indicates an atrial septal defect
   b) In right ventricle reflecting a ventricular septal defect, or
   c) In pulmonary arteries due to a patent ductus arteriosus.
3 Pressure studies: an increased pressure gradient between two communicating chambers indicates an intervening stenosis, e.g. high pressure in right ventricle and low pressure in pulmonary artery indicates pulmonary stenosis.
4 Indicator dilution techniques provide great accuracy in detecting the existence and location of right to left shunts. The standard technique of measuring flow in congenital heart disease is by the Fick method:

$$\text{Cardiac output (l/min)} = \frac{O_2 \text{ consumption (ml/min)}}{\text{A-V } O_2 \text{ difference (ml/min)}}$$

Cardiac embryology

The primitive heart and great vessels commence as symmetrical endocardial tubes. These primitive tubes fuse to form a single tubular heart which develops within the mesodermal cardiogenic plate surrounded by its myoepicardial mantle, which develops specific grooves demarcating, from before backward, a) the sinus venosus, b) the atrium, c) the ventricle, d) the bulbus cordis, e) truncus arteriosus.

With enlargement of the primitive tube it loses its symmetric contour, undergoing a tortuous bend to the left so that its distal end, which receives venous blood via the sinus venosus, comes to lie behind its proximal cephalic end with its large arteries. As it extends into the pericardial cavity, the dorsal mesentery breaks down to form the transverse sinus: a recess between the aorta and pulmonary artery posteriorly and the superior vena cava and left atrium anteriorly (Fig. 17.3).

The right part of the sinus venosus receives the major portion of the venous blood via the ductus venosus and is gradually absorbed into the atrium. The left part of the sinus venosus, which receives the pulmonary venous drainage, is similarly absorbed into the atrium.

Endocardial cushions develop dorsally and ventrally between the atrium and ventricle, narrowing the atrioventricular orifice and developing into atrioventricular valves (mitral and tricuspid).

The bulbus cordis is gradually incorporated into the ventricle, with disappearance of the ridge between these two components.

Longitudinal spiral cushions within the bulbus and the truncus arteriosus fuse to form a single spiral septum. This septum separates the left ventricular vestibule from the right ventricular infundibulum proximally and the aorta from the pulmonary trunk distally.

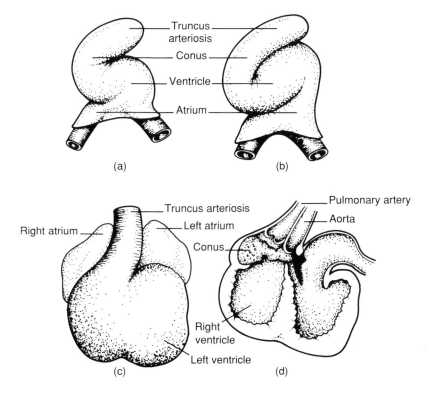

Fig. 17.3. Development of the heart.

Further Reading

Feigenbaum H. *Echocardiography.* 4th ed. Lea and Febiger. Philadelphia. 1986.

Fink B. W. *Congenital heart disease.* Year Book Medical Publishers Inc. Chicago. 1980.

Friedman H. H. *Outline of electrocardiography.* McGraw-Hill Book Co. Inc. New York. 1983.

Kisslo J., Adams D. B. (Eds). *An introduction to Doppler echocardiography.* Vols 1-4. Medicine Productions. New York. 1987.

Marks C. *Applied surgical anatomy.* Charles C. Thomas Publishers. Springfield. 1972.

Nadas A. S., Fyler D. C. *Pediatric cardiology.* 3rd ed. W. B. Saunders Co. Philadelphia. 1972.

Perry S. B., Keane J. F., Lock J. E. Interventional catheterization in pediatric congenital and acquired heart disease. *Am. J. Cardiol.* 61: 1090, 1988.

Chapter 18
Atrial Septal Defects

Embryology

Between the fourth and sixth week of gestation the primitive single-chambered atrium with its atrioventricular endocardial cushions is divided into right and left atria by a series of partitions that normally leave a transitory communication between right and left atria – the foramen ovale. This opening permits the fetal flow of oxygenated umbilical vein blood to flow through the inferior vena cava to the right atrium and reach the left atrium. Functional closure of the foramen ovale occurs soon after birth as pulmonary aeration increases left atrial pressure.

Even if the foramen remains patent (in 25% of adults) it is generally not functionally significant. Should there be a rise in right atrial pressure, e.g. pulmonary stenosis, then functional patency of the foramen will ensue, with shunting of blood from right to left atrium. Rarely is the shunt sufficient to cause cyanosis.

Septum primum: A crescentic partition grows cranio-caudally to reach the endocardial cushions, leaving a gap at the inferior margin – the ostium primum. As the septum primum then fuses with the endocardial cushions, the ostium primum is normally obliterated. The cranial end of the septum primum then thins and breaks down as a perforation to produce the ostium secundum.

Septum secundum: A second partition develops to the right of the septum primum, to form the septum secundum, and overlaps and obliterates the ostium secundum.

Defective absorption of the sinus venosus and pulmonary veins into the primitive atrium may lead to anomalous drainage of the pulmonary veins into the right atrium.

Clinical types

1 *Ostium secundum defects*: This defect is the most common variety of atrial septal defect (90%). It does not reach the atrioventricular valves and is situated behind the coronary sinus. The left to right shunt results in pulmonary blood flow greater than twice systemic flow. The defect is usually more than 2 cm in diameter so that future symptoms are inevitable (Fig. 18.1).

A systolic precordial murmur is associated with radiological evidence of pulmonary hilar hyperaemia and progressive development of right atrial enlargement. Clinical, radiological, electrocardiographic and echocardiographic examination will establish the diagnosis. If cardiac catheterization is carried out, an increased oxygen saturation at the atrial level will be noted.

The defect can be readily repaired either by direct suture or by application of a dacron patch after placing the patient on total cardiopulmonary bypass and opening the right atrium.

2 *Ostium primum defect*: The atrial defect is situated in the medial part of the septum in front of the coronary sinus. It is bounded medially by the junction of the tricuspid and mitral components

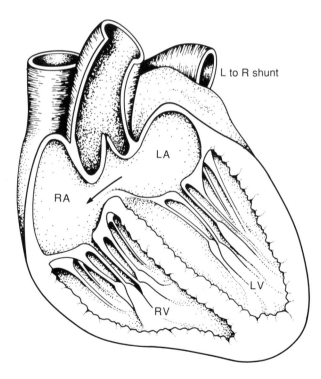

Fig. 18.1. Diagrammatic view of atrial septal defect.

of the atrioventricular valve on the crest of the underlying ventricular septum. Rarely existing alone, the failure of fusion between the septum primum and endocardial cushions is associated with:

a) Cleft mitral valve: there is a cleft in the aortic leaflet of the mitral valve. Abnormal chordae tendinae tether the cleft edges to the ventricular septum and may thereby maintain valvular competence despite the cleft. Severe mitral regurgitation may, however, cause serious haemodynamic problems with recurrent respiratory infections, dyspnoea and arrhythmia. A loud, harsh holosystolic murmur is audible to auscultation. Left axis deviation is noted electrocardiographically with prolongation of the PR interval. Chest X-ray reveals significant left atrial enlargement.

Echocardiography provides excellent information regarding ventricular and mitral valve function but angiography may be necessary to detail the degree of mitral insufficiency and to demonstrate the "gooseneck" narrowing of the left ventricular outflow tract due to the abnormal mitral cusp (Fig. 18.2).

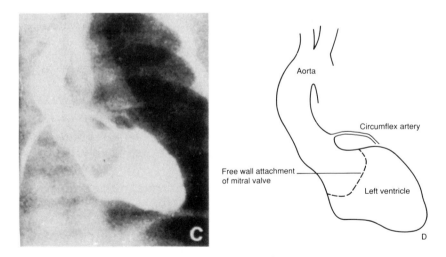

Fig. 18.2. "Gooseneck" narrowing of left ventricular outflow tract. C Angiographic view. D Diagrammatic view.

b) The tricuspid and mitral valve are cleft.
c) Complete atrioventricular canal: ostium primum defects are part of the spectrum of endocardial cushion defects which include the complete A-V canal.

3 *Sinus venosus defects*: These result from failed absorption of the sinus venosus into the right atrium. The defect is high on the septum with drainage of the right pulmonary veins into the superior vena cava. The right pulmonary veins may drain into the right atrium in association with all the varieties of atrial septal defect.

4 *Associated syndromes*
a) Lutembacher syndrome: this is represented by an ostium secundum atrial septal defect in association with congenital or acquired mitral stenosis. A large left to right shunt occurs because of flow impedance across the mitral valve. Elevation of jugular vein pressure and marked left atrial enlargement occur because of the mitral obstruction. Mitral valve calcification may develop. Atrial fibrillation often develops.
b) Marfan's syndrome
c) Noonan's syndrome: pulmonary valvular dysplasia causing pulmonary stenosis with small stature, hypertelorism, mild mental retardation, skeletal abnormalities, ptosis and crypt-orchidism
d) Holt–Oram syndrome: atrio-digital dysplasia: ostium secundum defect with maldevelopment or absence of thumb and radio-ulnar deformities.

General clinical manifestations
Atrial septal defects occur more commonly in females than males and patients are usually asymptomatic and rarely develop heart failure.

Haemodynamically, blood is shunted through the defect from left to right atrium. The increased blood flow to the right heart leads gradually to enlargement of the right atrium and right ventricle. There is greatly increased blood flow to the lungs with dilatation of the pulmonary arteries.

The presence of a systolic ejection murmur, best heard at the second left interspace, is attributable to an increased volume of blood ejected through the pulmonary valve during ventricular systole. There is wide splitting of the second sound due to delay in closure of the pulmonary valve.

The presence of right ventricular hypertrophy is indicative of an ostium secundum lesion, while an ostium primum lesion will demonstrate features consistent with left ventricular hypertrophy with left axis deviation on the electrocardiogram.

Though asymptomatic, patients are usually smaller in stature than normal, with a prominent left precordium and right ventricular enlargement radiologically and electrocardiographically in association with the systolic murmur.

The development of marked pulmonary hypertension with reversal of shunt flow is a very late phenomenon and is rarely encountered in the paediatric age range.

Complications
1 Congestive cardiac failure
2 Recurrent respiratory infections
3 Subacute bacterial endocarditis
4 Pulmonary hypertension: the development of right to left shunt will lead to pulmonary hypertension and cyanosis simulating the Eisenmenger syndrome
5 Paradoxical embolism: an embolus from the peripheral venous system may reach the left heart via a septal defect with systemic embolization.

Prognosis
In order to prevent effects later in life, despite the rarity of complications and the long delay before congestive cardiac failure occurs, surgical closure should be recommended and optimally carried out when the child is about 6 years of age.

Surgical treatment
Total cardiopulmonary bypass is established via a median sternotomy. The left ventricle is vented through the right superior pulmonary vein; the aorta is cross-clamped and cold cardioplegia standstill accomplished. The right atrium is opened anterior to the sulcus terminalis.

Ostium secundum defect

The secundum defect is located in the fossa ovalis region. Small defects may be closed by direct continuous suture, but larger defects should be closed with a patch.

Although a dacron or Gore-tex patch may be used, autogenous pericardium, hardened by 6 minutes of immersion in 0.6% glutaraldehyde, is preferable.

The patch is secured with continuous 4-0 prolene suture. Commencing at the superior margin of the defect, each end of the double-needled suture is brought down the sides of the defect and tied at the inferior margin. If the inferior margin is indistinct, the patch is secured to the atrial wall at its junction with the inferior vena cava. The right atrial incision is closed with 4-0 prolene suture and all air evacuated from the right atrium and pulmonary artery.

Final de-airing is accomplished by the cardioplegia needle in the aortic root, with removal of the aortic cross-clamp, while the heart is beating but not yet ejecting.

Lutembacher syndrome

The mitral valve is assessed and enlarged by commissurotomy before closing the atrial septal defect.

Sinus venosus defect

The right atrial incision is extended to the superior vena cava and the anatomy of the anomalous venous drainage is assessed. A pericardial patch is used to close the defect so that the anomalous pulmonary venous drainage is routed into the left atrium.

One should avoid narrowing the superior vena cava by use of a prosthetic patch or a flap of the right atrial appendage. The right atrium is then closed; the heart is de-aired and the operation concluded.

Ostium primum defect

As a partial form of endocardial cushion defect with an associated mitral cleft, suture repair of the cleft with 4-0 dacron suture will be necessary to prevent mitral regurgitation.

After the right atrium has been opened, the septal defect will be visualized between the tricuspid and mitral valves. An associated foramen ovale or secundum defect may also need closure.

The mitral cleft is repaired and valve competence assessed by injecting saline solution into the left ventricle via the vent. This will close the mitral leaflets. If a regurgitant jet persists, an annuloplasty may become necessary.

In closing the primum defect with a patch damage to the conduction system should be avoided by appropriately placed 4-0 prolene sutures.

The conducting system is located at the apex of the triangle of Koch and extends beneath the valve tissue to the left of the ventricular septum, continuing beyond the cleft mitral septal leaflet. The branching bundle then extends along the inferior margin of membranous septum, dividing into right and left bundles which continue into the ventricular sinuses. The right bundle then enters the anterolateral papillary muscle.

To avoid conduction bundle injury, interrupted 4-0 prolene sutures are placed superficially, staying to the right between the two atrioventricular valves. The sutures are positioned parallel to the flow of the conduction fibres to reduce the hazard of damage.

At the coronary sinus, the sutures are placed to the left of the coronary sinus valve and continue to the left of the tendon of Todaro.

Once this hazardous area has been negotiated, continuous 4-0 prolene can be used to complete the attachment of the rest of the patch to the free margin of the atrial septal defect.

After closure of the right atrium, temporary pacing wires are attached to the epicardium and brought out to the surface in case postoperative pacing is required.

Further Reading

Bull C., Deanfield J., de Laval M., Stark J. et al. Correction of isolated secundum atrial septal defect in infancy. Arch. Dis. Child 56: 784, 1981.

Keith J. D. In: Keith J. D., Rowe R. D. (Eds), Heart disease in infancy and childhood. 3rd edition. Macmillan. New York. 1978.

Kirklin J. W. and Barratt-Boyes B. G. Cardiac surgery. John Wiley and Sons. New York. 1986.

Spencer F. C. In: Sabiston D. C. Jnr, Spencer F. C. (Eds), Gibbons surgery of the chest. W. B. Saunders Co. Philadelphia. 1990.

Chapter 19
Ventricular Septal Defects

Atrial septal defects, ventricular septal defects and atrioventricular canal defects are different anomalies that share the commonality of representing intracardiac shunts.

Ventricular septal defect is a developmental cardiac abnormality that affects two children per 1000 live births. It may exist as the sole lesion or be associated with other congenital cardiac anomalies (Fig. 19.1).

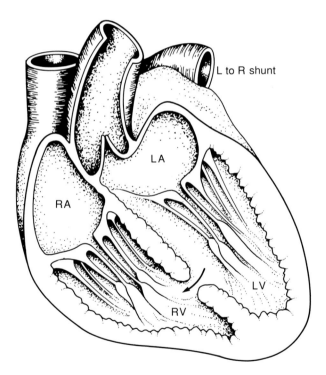

Fig. 19.1. Ventricular septal defect.

The defect may be categorized as being small or large. The small defects may cause little in the way of haemodynamic disturbance and the asymptomatic child will evidence a systolic murmur and thrill in the third left interspace and may be categorized as having "maladie de Roger".

Embryology

Three separate components undergo fusion, between the fourth and eighth weeks of gestation, to form the ventricular septum which divides the single ventricular chamber into two:

1 A primitive interventricular septum, destined to become the muscular septum, grows cephalad as the ventricular chambers enlarge, eventually meeting with the right and left ridges of the bulbus cordis. The right ridge fuses with the tricuspid valve and the endocardial cushion, thereby separating the tricuspid and pulmonary valves. The left ridge fuses with a ridge of the interventricular septum, leaving the aortic and mitral rings in continuity. The developing endocardial cushions fuse with the bulbar ridges and the muscular component of the septum.

2 Downgrowth from the endocardial cushions: a downgrowth from the right side of the atrioventricular cushion becomes the membranous septum and fuses distally with the muscular septum. The upper part of the partition separates the left ventricle from the right atrium because, as the septum straightens and elongates, the mitral valve becomes attached at a higher septal level than the tricuspid valve.

3 The bulbar septum: a bulbo-spiral partition or septum grows downwards from the truncus arteriosus to fuse with the membranous and muscular septa at the crista supra-ventricularis. Proximally the septum separates the infundibulum of the right ventricle from the vestibule of the left ventricle. Distally it divides the truncus arteriosus into pulmonary trunk and aortic root.

Types of defect(Fig. 19.2)

1 *Supracristal*: The deficiency is located above the crista supraventricularis. Situated immediately below the aortic and pulmonary valve annuli, it represents a defect in the bulbar

septum. Prolapse of the right aortic cusp into the septal opening
may cause aortic regurgitation. Occasionally mild right ventricular outflow tract obstruction develops.

2 *Membranous*: This is the commonest ventricular septal defect
(80%). There is a deficiency below the tricuspid valve. The
Bundle of His passes along the inferior margin of the defect on
the left ventricular aspect. This fact requires that great care be
taken in the insertion of sutures in this area. There may, rarely,
be an associated perforation in the tricuspid valve providing
haemodynamic changes similar to those in the Gerbode defect.

3 *The canal type*: The defect is situated more posteriorly in the
membranous septum where atrioventricular canal defects occur.

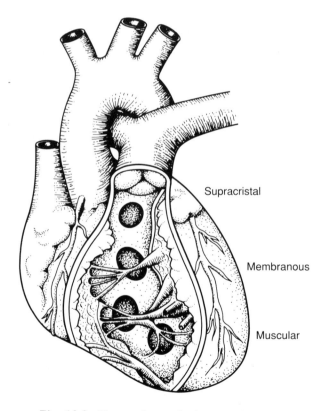

Supracristal

Membranous

Muscular

Fig. 19.2. Types of ventricular septal defects.

There is great surgical hazard to injury of the A-V node or the Bundle of His.

4 *Muscular defects*: The defects may be single or multiple and are often low in the septum. Muscular defect may also complicate cardiac trauma or myocardial infarction.

5 *Gerbode defect*: The communication is between left ventricle and right atrium. The defect is in the membranous septum above the tricuspid valve and blood flow from left ventricle to right atrium causes serious haemodynamic sequelae.

Haemodynamic effects

Small defects with small shunts are generally associated with normal pulmonary vascular resistance (Maladie de Roger). These may close spontaneously within the early years of life.

Large defects with large left to right shunts and normal pulmonary vascular resistance are amenable to surgical repair. A large defect allows equalization of pressure in both ventricles, leading to pressure and volume overload of the right ventricle. If pulmonary resistance remains low, blood flow will preferentially pass into the pulmonary artery rather than the aorta. This increased flow not only burdens the right heart, but the increased return of blood to the left atrium and left ventricle produces left ventricular overload with ultimate biventricular congestive heart failure.

As pulmonary vascular resistance increases it may exceed systemic resistance. There is reversal of blood flow with development of right to left shunt with ensuing central cyanosis and finger clubbing. This condition represents the Eisenmenger complex.

Clinical features

Most cases are first seen in the first and second decades. Uncomplicated ventricular septal defect is usually discovered in an asymptomatic, acyanotic child with a harsh, loud pansystolic murmur, and an accompanying palpable thrill, at the left 3rd or 4th interspace. There is a split second sound.

The pulse and blood pressure are normal. The heart may be normal in size or moderately enlarged.

The electrocardiogram may be normal but with significant shunts there may be features of left or bilateral ventricular hypertrophy.

Radiological examination of the chest is normal in mild cases but significant changes may be noted:

1 Pulmonary artery dilation and hilar hyperaemia. The hilar dance may be seen at fluoroscopy, but is not as prominent as in atrial septal defect.

2 Enlargement of left ventricle and atrium or of both ventricles.

Echocardiography will demonstrate the size and site of the defect, while colour flow Doppler will provide information regarding degree of shunting and blood flow.

Cardiac catheterization and angiography are now rarely necessary but will identify the site of the defect and permit measurement of oxygen saturation, with elevated levels in the right ventricle and pulmonary artery. Pressure studies may demonstrate increased pressure in the right ventricle and pulmonary artery. Calculation by the Fick formula from oxygen saturation levels will indicate the magnitude of the shunt.

Unless the patient is asymptomatic with a small or closing defect, surgical closure of the defect is recommended because of the possibility of serious complications. The spontaneous closure of ventricular septal defects will occur in 30% of small defects within 2 years and up to 50% within 10 years, thus careful follow-up and evaluation is warranted in asymptomatic children without complications. A large ventricular septal defect with pulmonary to systemic blood flow greater than 2 to 1 is a strong indication for surgical closure if: a) symptoms develop, b) pulmonary artery pressure is elevated, c) cardiac enlargement is present.

Complications

1 Development of congestive heart failure: usually with defects greater than 1.5 cm in diameter, developing in infancy or early childhood before the age of 2 years.

2 Progression to irreversible pulmonary hypertension: the defect is usually 1.5 – 3 cm in diameter and is not originally associated with the Eisenmenger complex.

3 Bacterial endocarditis is a rare complication but may affect small to moderate sized defects.

4 The development of infundibular hypertrophy and stenosis of the right ventricle converting large ventricular septal defects (1.5 – 3 cm) into Tetralogy of Fallot.

Medical treatment: The prophylaxis of bacterial endocarditis and management of cardiac failure remain the basis of non-operative management.

Surgical management
Repair of a ventricular septal defect requires awareness of the important identifiable anatomic landmarks of the region which include:
1   The medial border of the tricuspid valve ring
2   The outflow tract of the right ventricle situated between the tricuspid annulus and the pulmonary valve
3   The crista supraventricularis: this prominent muscular band extends along the floor of the outflow tract
4   The papillary muscle of the conus: arising from the interventricular septum, its chordae tendinae insert into the adjacent borders of the septal and anterior tricuspid leaflets. It is generally situated inferior to the membranous defect, though large defects may extend distal to the muscle.

   The left ventricular outflow tract can be seen through a large defect to lie behind and distal to the right outflow tract.

   The right and non-coronary cusps of the aortic valve can be seen through the defect and the papillary muscle of the conus is closely related.

   A supracristal defect is situated between the crista supraventricularis and the pulmonary valve in close proximity to the pulmonary valve and left cusp of the aortic valve.

   The defect may be located in the posterior segment of the septum beneath the septal leaflet of the tricuspid valve, usually as part of an A-V canal defect.

The conduction system
The atrioventricular node is situated at the apex of the triangle of Koch, which is bounded by:
1   The coronary sinus, forming the base of the triangle
2   The tricuspid valve annulus
3   The tendon of Todaro.

   The Bundle of His passes through the central fibrous body into the interventricular septum, located at the inferior border of the membranous septum on its left side.

It gives off the fasciculi of the posterior radiation of the left bundle branch and at its bifurcation divides into the right bundle and the anterior radiation of the left bundle branch.

The right bundle branch passes to the right side of the septum and reaches the moderator band, i.e. the anterolateral papillary muscle. Conduction fibres do not extend beyond the papillary muscle of the conus.

Repair of perimembranous ventricular septal defect

Transatrial approach

This is the preferred approach, especially in infants. Ventricular function is preserved by avoiding a ventriculotomy.

Via a midline sternotomy, total cardiopulmonary bypass and cardioplegic cardiac arrest are performed in standard fashion. The right atrium is opened widely anterior to the sulcus terminalis. If an associated foramen ovale or secundum atrial defect is found, it will be closed.

Retraction of the septal leaflet of the tricuspid valves exposes the ventricular defect. A dacron patch is tailored and the defect closed using interrupted teflon-pledgeted 4-0 ticron sutures. The sutures passing through the base of the tricuspid leaflet do not need pledget reinforcement.

The atriotomy is closed, the heart is de-aired and decannulated in standard fashion and the operation concluded.

Transventricular approach

The right ventricle is incised transversely, avoiding injury to coronary artery branches. The Bundle of His lies on the left ventricular side of the septum, requiring that all septal sutures posterior to the papillary muscle of the conus should be placed as interrupted mattress sutures 2-3 mm from the edge of the right ventricular side of the septum.

If the tricuspid valve lines the posterior border of the defect, the sutures should be passed through the base of the tricuspid valve. Any gap between the tricuspid valve and the septal wall is closed by a transitional suture that passes between the right side of the septal muscle, through the tricuspid leaflet at the valve annulus, into the atrium and then back through the valve tissue to the ventricle.

Beyond the papillary muscle of the conus, it is safe to take full-thickness bites without endangering the conducting bundle. At the upper margin of the defect, suture placement should avoid injury to the aortic valve.

Alternatively, continuous sutures can be used to close most of the defect, interrupted sutures being used, however, at the transitional zone (Fig. 19.3).

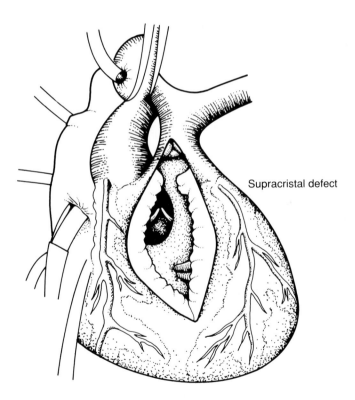

Supracristal defect

Fig. 19.3. Supracristal VSD due to failed fusion between bulbar ridges, endocardial cushions and muscular septum.

The ventriculotomy can usually be closed by a double row of 4-0 prolene sutures, but if there is risk of narrowing the pulmonary outflow tract, closure may be accomplished by a pericardial patch as in reconstruction of Tetralogy of Fallot.

Repair of a muscular defect

Muscular defects in the trabecular septum may be multiple with a "Swiss-cheese" appearance.

An incision at the apex of the left ventricle is made parallel to the left anterior descending artery, exposing the anteriorly placed lesion. Although the defect has multiple openings on the right side, there is a single opening if viewed from the left ventricle.

The rim of the defect is free of any conductile fibres, permitting closure of the defect by a patch sutured in continuous fashion with 4-0 prolene. The left ventriculotomy is closed and the operation concluded in the standard manner.

Pulmonary artery banding

This procedure is used to reduce pulmonary artery pressure to normal physiological levels i.e. 30–50% of systemic pressure. It may be indicated in infants, as a palliative measure, to reduce excessive pulmonary blood flow associated with large left to right intracardiac shunts, e.g. ventricular septal defects; A-V canal; truncus arteriosus.

This closed operation is performed via a left anterior 3rd interspace thoracotomy. The pericardium is opened anterior to the phrenic nerve. The pulmonary artery is dissected free and a 5 mm wide woven teflon tape is passed round it and tightened until the mean pulmonary artery pressure is half to one-third of mean systemic pressure. The tape is secured with several interrupted sutures.

Subsequent removal of the band will be done at the time of total correction of the lesion via a midline sternotomy.

The tissue overlying the band is incised on each side of the sutured area and removed. The central band with the incorporated pulmonary artery tissue is excised and the controlled pulmonary artery defect is closed with a patch of autologous tissue. The patient is then placed on cardiopulmonary bypass and the definitive procedure carried out.

Further Reading

Hoffman J. I. E., Rudolph A. M. The natural history of isolated ventricular septal defect with special reference to selection as patients for surgery. *Adv. Pediatr.* 17: 57, 1970.

Kirklin J. K., Castaneda A. R., Keane J. F. *et al.* Surgical management of multiple ventricular septal defects. *J. Thorac. Cardiovasc. Surg.* 80: 485, 1980.

Lincoln C., Jamieson S., Joseph M. *et al.* Transatrial repair of ventricular septal defects with reference to their anatomic classification. *J. Thorac. Cardiovasc. Surg.* 74: 183, 1977.

Chapter 20
Complete Atrioventricular Canal

Persistence of a common atrioventricular (A-V) canal may cause a range of cardiac malformations which involve, singly or in combination, the atrial septum, the ventricular septum and one or both atrioventricular valves (Fig. 20.1).

Synonyms
Endocardial cushion defect; canalis atrioventricularis communis; persistent A-V ostium.

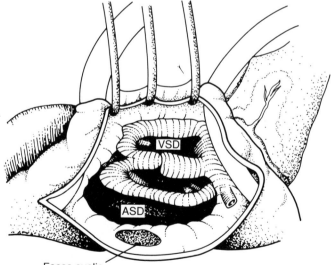

Fig. 20.1. Complete A-V canal: operative view.

Embryology
The malformations result from defective development of one or more of the following structures:
1 The atrial septum with persistence of the ostium primum
2 The ventral and dorsal endocardial cushions
3 The ventricular septum: deficiency of the membranous septum and the inferior portion of the conus septum.

Type
Incomplete forms
1 Without interventricular communication:
   a) Ostium primum atrial septal defect and cleft mitral valve
   b) Common atrium with A-V valve deformity
   c) Isolated ostium primum defect or cleft mitral or cleft tricuspid valve.
2 With interventricular communication:
   a) Ventricular septal defect of A-V canal type; normal A-V valves
   b) VSD of A-V canal type + abnormal A-V valves.

Complete forms
1 *Type I*: With divided, septally attached ventral common leaflet
2 *Type II*: With divided, septally unattached ventral common leaflet
3 *Type III*: With undivided, septally unattached ventral common leaflet.

Clinical features
The condition is common in children with trisomy 21 (Down's syndrome). The child fails to thrive and is underweight.

Tachycardia and tachypnoea are present and the precordium is prominent and hyperactive. The child suffers recurrent respiratory infections and congestive heart failure develops within 2 months of birth, with hepatomegaly, ascites and distended neck veins.

The child with an endocardial cushion defect has the potential for blood flow between any of the four cardiac chambers, with corresponding increase in size of all the chambers leading to gross cardiomegaly and marked increase in pulmonary vascularity resulting from the left to right shunt.

Although there is often a characteristic harsh pansystolic murmur, an associated diastolic rumble may reflect the large left to right shunt. At times, however, a balanced intracardiac haemodynamic status is attained with minimal shunting and absence of a murmur.

Electrocardiography reveals left axis deviation associated with right bundle branch block. Features of biventricular hypertrophy may be noted.

Radiological examination of the chest will demonstrate gross cardiomegaly and increased pulmonary vascularity.

2-D echocardiography reveals a common A-V valve associated with a large high-lying ventricular septal defect and a low-lying, ostium primum, atrial septal defect.

With cardiac catheterization, the catheter may pass into all four chambers in a bizarre manner. A large left to right shunt and rapidly developing pulmonary hypertension is revealed. The pulmonary hypertension may become irreversible within 12–24 months.

Angiography will define the typical "goose-neck" deformity of the left ventricular outflow tract due to the abnormal attachment of the mitral valve to the septum (Fig. 20.2).

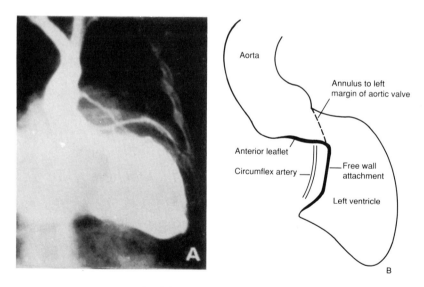

Fig. 20.2. Complete A-V canal:
A Angiographic appearance.   B Diagrammatic representation.

Techniques of surgical repair

1 *Two patch technique:* This is the preferred technique as there is no need to incise the ventral and dorsal leaflets and there will be no risk of their separation at their attachments to the patches.
2 *One patch technique.*
3 *Banding of the pulmonary artery* is reserved for infants less than 4 months old with severe heart failure unresponsive to medical measures. Total repair is recommended whenever possible within 2 years.

A midline sternotomy provides access for total cardiopulmonary bypass and hypothermic, cardioplegic arrest. The right atrium is opened anterior to the sulcus terminalis.

The anatomical details of the defects and of the valve leaflets are studied. If the ventral and dorsal leaflets are undivided, they are incised along the right atrial side at the ventricular septal plane. The mitral component should be left with enough tissue to provide competence of the reconstructed mitral valve.

The edges of the ventral and dorsal leaflets are approximated and the cleft in the mitral valve septal leaflet is repaired with several interrupted 4-0 prolene sutures.

Two patch technique

1 A dacron prosthesis is sutured into the ventricular septal defect. Mattress sutures of 4-0 prolene are used to appose the top of this patch to the ventral and dorsal leaflets.
2 A pericardial patch is sutured into the atrial defect and mattress sutures at the edges of the valve leaflet are used to appose them to the pericardial patch.

Single patch technique

An appropriate-sized patch of dacron or autologous pericardium is sutured to the right ventricular side of the septum with 4-0 pledgeted ticron sutures, either as mattress or continuous sutures.

The septal leaflet of the mitral valve is attached to the patch with 4-0 ticron mattress sutures which pass through the mitral leaflet, the patch and the cut edge of the tricuspid leaflet.

With the leaflets attached to the patch, mitral valve competence is tested by injecting saline into the left ventricle. If incompetence persists, complete suturing of cleft, annuloplasty or shortening of chordae tendinae may be carried out.

The upper end of the patch is then used to close the atrial septal defect by continuous 4-0 ticron suture.

The right atrium is closed, the heart de-aired and decannulated and the operation concluded in standard manner.

Further Reading

Berger T. J., Kirklin J. W., Blackstone E. H. *et al.* Primary repair of complete atrioventricular canal in patients less than 2 years old. *Am. J. Cardiol.* 41: 906, 1978.

Piccoli, G. P., Wilkinson J. L., Macartney F. J. *et al.* Morphology and classification of complete atrio-ventricular defects. *Br. Heart J.* 46: 633, 1979.

Rastelli G. C., Ongley P. A., Kirklin J. W., McGoon D. C. Surgical repair of the complete form of persistent common atrio-ventricular canal. *J. Thorac. Cardiovasc. Surg.* 55: 299, 1968.

Chapter 21
Patent Ductus Arteriosus

The ductus arteriosus is an anatomical structure derived embryologically from the 6th branchial arch. It connects the left pulmonary artery to the isthmus of the descending thoracic aorta. The ductus normally closes physiologically within 24 hours of birth, but anatomic obliteration takes several weeks (Fig. 21.1).

Although a patent ductus usually exists as an isolated abnormality, it may coexist with other cardiovascular anomalies, e.g. coarctation of the aorta.

It may function as an important compensatory channel in

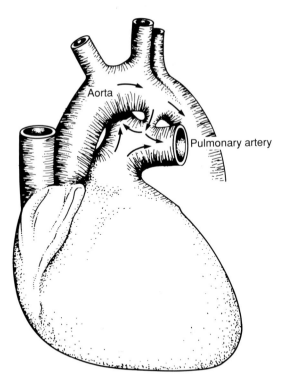

Fig. 21.1. Patent ductus arteriosus.

Tetralogy of Fallot, tricuspid atresia or transposition of the great arteries. The oral administration of prostaglandins will prolong the patency of the channel in the neonatal period in babies with such cyanotic heart anomalies.

Patent ductus arteriosus represents the most common of the extracardiac shunts, the others being:
1 Aortico-pulmonary septal defect
2 Anomalous pulmonary venous drainage
3 Pulmonary arteriovenous fistula
4 Rupture of sinus of Valsalva aneurysm into right atrium.

Fetal circulation
The umbilical vein channels oxygenated blood through the inferior vena cava to the right atrium. Blood flow is deflected through the foramen ovale to the left atrium, courses into the left ventricle and via the aorta to the brachiocephalic arteries.

The brachiocephalic venous return courses through the right atrium to the right ventricle and then through the pulmonary artery. The high pulmonary vascular resistance in the collapsed airless lungs causes most of the blood flow to pass through the patent ductus arteriosus to the descending aorta, providing less oxygenated blood to the lower body.

Post-natal circulation
With the first inspiratory pulmonary inflation at birth, there is a marked reduction in pulmonary vascular resistance and the pressure in the pulmonary artery falls below that in the aorta, inducing closure of the ductus.

Should the ductus remain patent, the flow through it will be from aorta to pulmonary artery. By increasing the total pulmonary blood flow, there will be an increased load on the left atrium and left ventricle.

Rarely pulmonary vascular resistance remains high after birth, resulting in patent ductus arteriosus with pulmonary hypertension. As unsaturated pulmonary artery blood flows to the aortic isthmus below the brachio-cephalic arteries, differential cyanosis will affect the lower limbs only. The presence of irreversible pulmonary hypertension contraindicates surgical closure of the ductus.

Clinical features

The volume overload on the left heart results from aortopulmonary flow through the ductal shunt as the aortic pressure is greater. Although a large left to right shunt may cause recurrent episodes of respiratory infection, dyspnoea and failure to thrive, usually the children are asymptomatic, the only overt clinical sign being the continuous "machinery" to-and-fro (Gibson) murmur in the infraclavicular and precordial area radiating to the back. There may be a large-amplitude, "waterhammer", collapsing pulse in association with a large ductus.

Apart from the neonate who may present with acute cardiac failure, diagnosis is usually established in the asymptomatic child during the first decade.

Symptoms may develop because of complications:

1 Congestive cardiac failure
2 Recurrent attacks of respiratory infection
3 Subacute bacterial endocarditis
4 Pulmonary hypertension

Diagnosis

Electrocardiography: The ECG will be normal in mild cases but if the shunt is large, left ventricular hypertrophy will be reflected in tall R waves in left ventricular leads (V5 and V6) and deep S waves in right ventricular leads (V1 and V2). Depression of ST segments and inversion of T waves in the left ventricular leads are indicative of left ventricular strain.

Chest roentgenography: Cardiomegaly due to left ventricular enlargement, prominence of the pulmonary conus and increased vascularity of the lung fields may be apparent. The aortic knuckle may be prominent. (Fig. 21.2).

Echocardiography: The amount of shunt flow and the direction of flow through the ductus arteriosus can be demonstrated by Doppler techniques. 2-D echocardiography can delineate the patent ductus.

Cardiac catheterization: Rarely necessary but if performed the catheter can be visualized passing from pulmonary artery through the patent ductus into the aorta.

The oxygen saturation in the pulmonary artery will be raised, and pressure in the pulmonary artery will be moderately increased if the shunt is large.

Angiocardiography may be done if the diagnosis is in doubt. A catheter is passed into the arch of the aorta via the femoral or brachial artery with delineation of the patent ductus by injected contrast material.

Treatment
Medical
Antibiotic therapy may be necessary in the prophylaxis of bacterial endocarditis during infection or operative procedures. In the

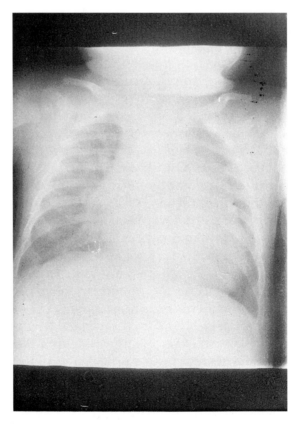

Fig. 21.2. Left ventricular enlargement, prominence of pulmonary conus and increased lung vascularity, due to longstanding PDA, viewed radiologically.

presence of infective endocarditis intensive antibiotic therapy precedes surgical ligation or division of the ductus.

Congestive cardiac failure may require preoperative management.

Indomethacin: The association of patent ductus arteriosus with neonatal respiratory distress syndrome in premature infants merits fluid restriction and administration of indomethacin. By inhibiting the production of prostaglandin synthesis, it may cause contraction of ductal tissue and cause its closure. If treatment fails, operation is indicated.

Surgical management

Although the presence of congestive heart failure may demand immediate ligation of a patent ductus arteriosus, the procedure can usually be delayed until the child is about 1 year of age.

Procedure

Under general inhalation anaesthetic, the child is placed in the right lateral decubitus position and a left 4th intercostal space thoracotomy performed. After placement of the rib spreader, the lung apex is retracted down and medially. The mediastinal pleura is opened over the aortic isthmus, continuing proximally along the left subclavian artery and distally below the isthmus. Finger palpation will experience a thrill maximally over the patent ductus. The superior intercostal vein will be identified, ligated and divided.

The dissection continues over the anterior surface of the aorta across the ductus towards the pulmonary artery. Identification of the left vagus nerve and its recurrent laryngeal nerve as it curves posteriorly round the ductus is now the key to mobilization of the ductus. The nerves are kept in view on the pulmonary artery side of the dissection to avoid their injury. The pericardial lappet extending over the anterior surface of the ductus is now mobilized and reflected medially (Fig. 21.3).

Tapes are placed around the mobilized aorta above and below the ductus and around the left subclavian artery, and vascular clamps are placed within reach in case haemorrhage occurs.

The dense tissue on the posterior wall of the ductus and the aortic isthmus is then carefully cleared with the knowledge that this can be the most critical and hazardous phase of the procedure.

1 *Division of the patent ductus arteriosus*: Vascular clamps are secured on either side of the ductus, as close as possible to the aorta and pulmonary artery respectively. After division of the ductus, with an adequate cuff of tissue extending beyond each clamp, each end is closed with continuous 6-0 prolene sutures. The pulmonary artery clamp is then removed first, followed by careful removal of the aortic clamp. Division of the ductus prevents the possibility of ductal recanalization.

2 *Ligation* of the patent ductus is recommended in the neonate and during the first year of life. In the neonate the ductus may be larger than the aortic arch and isthmus and appears to be in continuity with the descending aorta.

The ductus is exposed and cleared and a size 1 silk ligature is passed around the ductus and tied firmly enough to occlude the ductal lumen. If there is room, a second suture may be applied around the ductus.

Alternatively a 3-0 prolene purse-string suture may be placed on the aortic side, taking superficial bites of the aortic wall and a second ligature used on the pulmonary artery side.

PATENT DUCTUS ARTERIOSUS

CLINICAL ANATOMY:

(i) Patent channel between aortic asthmus and main or left pulmonary artery

(ii) Machinery murmur

(iii) Variable growth retardation

(iv) Complications:

(a) Pulmonary hypertension
(b) Cardiac Failure
(c) Subacute bacterial endocarditis

Fig. 21.3. Clinical anatomy of PDA.

In the neonate a large liga-clip can be used to occlude the ductus, thereby avoiding dissection of the posterior ductal wall.

3 *Calcified aneurysmal patent ductus arteriosus*: In older patients either calcification or aneurysmal enlargement increase the dangers of operation. A Gott shunt may be inserted through purse-string sutures in the aorta above and below the ductus, with blood flow continuing through the Gott shunt. The pulmonary side of the ductus is clamped and the ductus is opened. The pulmonary and aortic orifices of the ductus are oversewn and all clamps are removed, as is the Gott shunt with purse-string sutures tied.

4 *Associated complex cardiac abnormalities*: Via a midline sternotomy, cannulae are inserted in preparation for cardiopulmonary by-pass.

The ductus is dissected free and ligated, cardiopulmonary bypass instituted and the definitive procedures carried out.

If dissection of the ductus proves difficult, partial cardio-pulmonary bypass is instituted and the aorta is cross-clamped. The pulmonary artery is incised and the ductal orifice is sutured closed. The pulmonary arteriotomy is sutured and the definitive procedure carried out.

Further Reading

Brano B., Doty D. *et al.* Ligation of patent ductus arteriosus in premature infants. *Ann. Thorac. Surg.* 32: 167, 1981.

Gross R. E. The patent ductus arteriosus: Observations on diagnosis and therapy in 525 surgically treated cases. *Am. J. Med.* 12: 472, 1952.

Gross R. E., Hubbard J. P. Surgical ligation of a patent ductus arteriosus. *J.A.M.A.* 112: 729, 1939.

Mitchell J. R. A. Prostaglandins in vascular disease, a seminal approach. *Br. Med. J.* 282: 590, 1981.

Wernly J. A. Intra-aortic closure of the calcified patent ductus. *J. Thorac. Cardiovasc. Surg.* 80: 206, 1980.

Chapter 22
Aortopulmonary Window

A septal defect between the aorta and pulmonary artery is caused by maldevelopment during embryologic fusion of the conotruncal ridges and during the development of the pulmonary arteries from the right and left sixth aortic arches.

Types
1 The communication is situated between the ascending aorta and the main pulmonary artery, distal to their respective valves (Fig. 22.1).
2 The communication is at the bifurcation of the main pulmonary artery and the ascending aorta where it crosses the pulmonary artery.
3 The right pulmonary artery arises from the ascending aorta. This type is curable by detaching the right pulmonary artery from the aortic arch and re-anastomosing it to the main pulmonary artery.

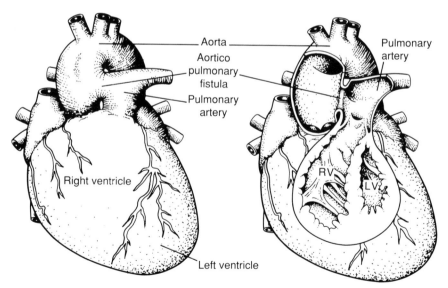

Fig. 22.1. Aorto-pulmonary window.

Clinical features
This rare defect clinically resembles a large patent ductus arteriosus
or large ventricular septal defect.
1 Congestive cardiac failure: infants present with feeding difficulties, failure to thrive, recurrent respiratory infections, tachycardia, tachypnoea and hepatomegaly.
2 Systolic ejection murmur or continuous murmur with bounding
   peripheral pulses and wide pulse pressure.
      Radiographic examination of the chest reveals cardiomegaly
   and increased pulmonary vascularity.
      Electrocardiography reflects either left ventricular or
   biventricular hypertrophy.
      2-D echocardiography will identify a defect between aorta
   and pulmonary artery. Its localization will be aided by colour
   Doppler flow techniques.
      Cardiac catheterization will confirm a left to right shunt but
   only aortography will establish an accurate diagnosis.

Surgical treatment
A midline sternotomy is performed and cardiopulmonary bypass
instituted. The aorta is cross-clamped, the aortic root is incised and
cardioplegia induced by perfusion through the coronary ostia. The
defect is visualized and a dacron patch sutured into the defect
with 4-0 prolene sutures. The aortotomy is closed and after de-
airing and removal of the aortic clamp, cardiopulmonary bypass is
discontinued and the procedure concluded.
   Circulatory arrest may be necessary for repair of Type I lesions,
so that the aortic cannula can be removed during repair of the
lesion.

Further Reading
Blieden L. C., Moller J. H. Aortopulmonary septal defect: An experience
   with 17 patients. *Br. Heart J.* 36: 630, 1974.
Doty D. B., Richardson J. V., Falkovsky G. E. *et al.* Aortopulmonary septal
   defect: Haemodynamics, angiography and operation. *Ann. Thorac. Surg.*
   32: 244, 1981.

Chapter 23
Coarctation of the Aorta

Coarctation of the aorta is a congenital narrowing of the aorta occurring just distal to the left subclavian artery. The aortic isthmus, between the left subclavian artery and the site of the ductus or ligamentum arteriosum, is the commonest site of constriction. The constriction is usually localized but may be elongated and tapered. Coarctation can, however, occur at any level along the course of the aorta, with occasional predilection for the abdominal aorta at the level of the renal arteries or the aortic arch.

Associated anomalies
Coarctation of the aorta is a common congenital anomaly, representing 8% of all causes of congenital heart disease. It is more common in males than females but is the most common cardiac abnormality in patients with Turner's syndrome. Although it usually exists as an isolated lesion, associated congenital cardiovascular conditions include patent ductus arteriosus, bicuspid aortic valve and subaortic or aortic stenosis. Aneurysms of the cerebral circle of Willis and extravascular malformations such as double vagina, cryptorchidism and polycystic or ectopic kidneys may coexist with coarctation.

Pathogenesis
It is unlikely that the overgrowth of tissue that normally causes closure of the ductus arteriosus can be a factor in its causation, as coarctation may be associated with a patent ductus or may occur some distance from the ligamentum arteriosum.

In embryonic life the subclavian arteries lie distal to the 6th aortic arch which gives rise to the ductus. With subsequent differential growth at the aortic isthmus, the subclavian arteries come to be proximal to the ductus. The altered position of the isthmus resulting from differential growth during embryonic life may result in redundant aortic tissue consolidating as a coarctation.

Types of coarctation

Aortic coarctation is best categorized by the associated patency or obliteration of the ductus arteriosus and may be defined (Fig. 23.1) as:

1 *Preductal coarctation*: This form, synonymous with the "infantile" type, is associated with early infant death in about 90% of cases because of severe strain on the right ventricle with right ventricular failure and lower extremity cyanosis. The pulmonary artery communicates with the distal thoracic aorta through the large patent ductus or other cardiac abnormality, such as atrial or ventricular septal defect or transposition of the great vessels. The left ventricular flow is routed to the brachiocephalic circulation, while the pulmonary artery flow is routed via the patent ductus to the lower body and limbs, thereby inhibiting the formation of a collateral intercostal circulation.

2 *Postductal coarctation*: The characteristic uncomplicated coarctation is located distal to the ductus or ligamentum arteriosum, with post-stenotic dilatation of the thoracic aorta. A bicuspid aortic valve is present in 25% of cases and may be associated with an early diastolic murmur due to aortic incompetence.

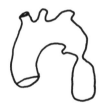

PREDUCTAL TYPES

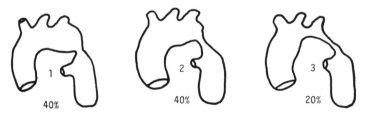

Scetches of representative types of coarctation. Percentages represent incidence of preductal types. Based on Keith et al (1958).

Fig. 23.1. Types of aortic coarctation.

A prominent collateral circulation develops between arteries proximal to the coarctation, such as internal mammary, subscapular, lateral thoracic and transverse scapular, which anastomose distally with the intercostal and inferior epigastric arteries which become markedly dilated, thin-walled and aneurysmal, often discernible clinically by their pulsation and visualized as rib notching on radiographic films of the chest (Fig. 23.2).

3 *Aortic atresia*: The interrupted aorta represents a most severe form of coarctation which is usually associated with a patent ductus arteriosus, often with other cardiac anomalies.

4 *Coarctation of the abdominal aorta*: This may represent an acquired middle-aortic syndrome with renovascular involvement as part of Takayasu's aortitis.

Clinical manifestations

The condition is more common in males. It may first present clinically in infancy with congestive heart failure that requires medical improvement followed by early corrective operation.

Systemic hypertension: The patient with coarctation may remain

COARCTATION OF AORTA

Clinical Anatomy

    i. Localised constriction
   ii. Bicuspid aortic valve (30% of cases)
  iii. Enlarged dilated collateral arteries:
        a. Internal mammary
        b. Intercostal
        c. Subscapular
        d. Lateral thoracic

   iv. Notching of ribs by collateral vessels
    v. Post-stenotic dilation
   vi. Effects of hypertension
  vii. Diminished arterial flow to lower limbs

Fig. 23.2. Clinical anatomy of aortic coarctation.

asymptomatic until the teens or early adulthood, when the effects of hypertension may become pronounced.

The blood pressure proximal to the constriction is increased, so that hypertension in the upper extremities is matched by reduced blood pressure in the lower extremities with decreased or absent pulses in the femoral arteries.

Diminished distal blood flow may result in impaired development of the lower body, cold feet and features of peripheral vascular inadequacy.

A precordial systolic ejection murmur is audible, radiating into cervical and mitral areas, and is often loudest posteriorly in the interscapular area.

Electrocardiography may reveal left ventricular hypertrophy and strain, but may be normal in patients with mild to moderate coarctation.

Radiographic examination
1 The heart may be normal in size or reveal cardiomegaly.
2 Rib notching: the pulsatile erosion of the anterior inferior margin or posterior segment of the 3rd to 8th ribs by enlarged collateral vessels rarely becomes apparent before 9 years of age.
3 The inverted "3" sign is caused by the intervening indentation between the dilated subclavian artery proximally and the post-stenotic dilatation of the aorta distally.
4 Indentation of the barium-filled oesophagus will be caused by poststenotic aortic dilatation (Fig. 23.3).
5 Aortography will provide an accurate preoperative diagnosis of the site and extent of the coarctation (Fig. 23.4).

Echocardiography
2-D echocardiography will define the coarcted segment and will identify associated cardiac anomalies.

The patient with coarctation may first present because of symptoms caused by complications:
1 Cardiac failure
2 Rupture of the aorta with sudden death, especially during parturition

3 Subacute bacterial endocarditis of a bicuspid valve or at the site of the constriction
4 Cerebral haemorrhage from the effects of hypertension or rupture of an associated cerebral aneurysm.

Surgical management

As only 25% of patients can anticipate living asymptomatically to an advanced age, surgical treatment is advised and, ideally, should be carried out between 2 and 6 years of age. Maximum growth of the aorta will have occurred, the vessel is pliable without atherosclerotic changes and the serious effects of systemic hypertension have not yet developed.

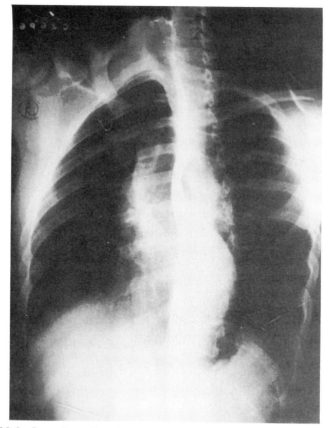

Fig. 23.3. Oesophageal indentation due to post-stenotic aortic dilation.

If cardiac failure occurs at an early age, aggressive medical therapy should be utilized and operation postponed to permit the aorta time to enlarge and sustain a larger blood flow, and thereby prevent subsequent restenosis at the anastomotic site. Delay beyond 10 years of age introduces the danger of aortic medial cystic necrosis, with increased operative hazard.

Excision of the coarctation

With the patient in the right lateral position, a left 4th interspace thoracotomy provides optimal access if the incision extends from a point anterior and inferior to the tip of the scapula proximally between scapula and vertebral spinous processes. Large, dilated

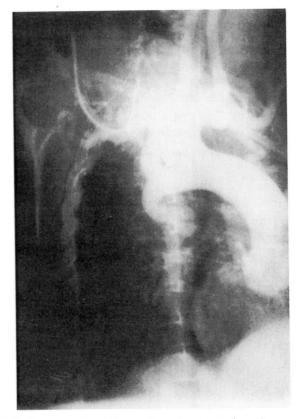

Fig. 23.4. Aortography defines site and extent of aortic coarctation.

collateral arteries in the subcutaneous, intermuscular and intercostal planes need to be ligated and divided to provide careful haemostasis. Entry into the pleural cavity permits retraction of the rib cage. The lung is retracted downwards and medially and the aortic isthmus exposed by opening the overlying mediastinal pleura.

The highest intercostal vein overlying the aorta is doubly ligated and divided, the fibroareolar tissue cleared to delineate the coarcted area as well as the left subclavian artery, adjacent poststenotic dilated aorta, the ductus or ligamentum arteriosus and the dilated intercostal arteries.

The ductus or ligamentum is isolated, doubly clamped and divided after identifying the vagus and left recurrent laryngeal nerves, which are kept unharmed. The divided ends of the patent ductus are oversewn with a continuous suture of 5-0 prolene while the divided ligamentum is tied with 2-0 silk.

The uppermost friable dilated intercostal arteries and bronchial arteries are carefully ligated with transfixion silk sutures and divided without use of clamps.

After mobilization, tapes are passed round the subclavian artery and the aorta above and below the constriction.

1 *Resection with end-to-end anastomosis*: Pott's clamps are placed across the aorta above and below the coarcted segment and temporary silk ties placed around the intercostal arteries that can be conserved. The coarcted segment is resected so that adequate proximal and distal lumina are available for anastomotic reconstruction.

   End-to-end anastomosis is accomplished with a posterior continuous everting suture of 4-0 prolene with intima to intima apposition. It is drawn taut and tied to an anchoring suture at each end. The anterior layer is completed as a series of interrupted everting sutures to prevent anastomotic constriction. The lower clamp is removed and the upper clamp slowly released.

   In infants interrupted mattress sutures of 4-0 vicryl or chromic catgut will reduce the prospect of anastomotic narrowing.

2 *Interposition graft*: An interposition graft of dacron or Gore-tex is inserted after excision of a long stenotic segment using 4-0

prolene suture. It is also indicated in older adults in whom arteriosclerotic and aneurysmal changes or post-stenotic dilation preclude an end-to-end anastomosis (Fig. 23.5).

3 *Aortoplasty*: In children in whom the upper aortic end is narrow and cone-shaped, the lumen may be enlarged by incising the aorta longitudinally; the internal luminal shelf is excised and a diamond-shaped plastic prosthesis sutured into place, permitting growth of the residual circumference.

This technique also has merit in children with re-coarctation.

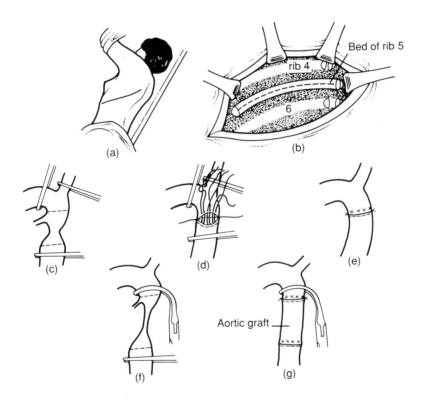

Fig. 23.5. Operative management of aortic coarctation.
A Incision.   B Subperiosteal rib resection.   C Sites of resection of coarctation.
D Aortic continuity restored with posterior running suture.
E Interrupted anterior sutures.   F Tubular coarctation.
G Interposed dacron graft.

4 *Subclavian flap*: In infants less than 1 year of age, older patients with re-coarctation, or in older children with a long coarcted segment this procedure has merit.

The subclavian artery is ligated at the origin of the vertebral artery, which is also ligated to prevent a subsequent steal syndrome, and is divided. After appropriate clamp control, an aortic incision begins distal to the constriction and extends proximally through the coarctation, isthmus and the subclavian artery. The coarcted luminal shelf is excised and the subclavian flap brought down to the aorta and sutured in place with 5-0 absorbable continuous suture.

The mediastinal pleura is resutured, a chest tube placed for drainage and the thoracotomy incision closed.

Postoperative complications

1 *Paraplegia*: This uncommon complication results from inadequate blood flow to the anterior spinal artery due to interruption of the intercostal collateral arteries. It is the patient with mild coarctation with minimal collateral development who is at greatest risk.

2 *Paradoxical hypertension*: In a third of young patients a marked rise in blood pressure may be noted postoperatively due to enhanced sympathetic activity. There is a good response to sympatholytic drugs.

3 *Mesenteric arteritis*: Abdominal pain, vomiting and fever are associated with generalized abdominal tenderness and ileus, at times progressing to intestinal gangrene that requires resection. The condition has an incidence of 5%.

4 *Recurrent coarctation*: with progressive fibrotic stenosis at the repair site. In view of the increased hazards, reoperation should be recommended only if:
   a) Symptoms of hypertension are severe
   b) The gradient is greater than 40 mm
   c) The diameter of the stenosed aorta is less than 55% that of the aorta at the diaphragm
   d) Congestive cardiac failure occurs.

Interrupted aortic arch

Congenital absence of the aortic arch is often accompanied by patency of the ductus arteriosus and presence of a ventricular septal defect:

Types

1 The interruption is distal to the left subclavian artery.
2 The interruption is between left carotid and left subclavian artery.
3 The interruption is between the innominate artery and the left common carotid artery.

Clinical features

Congestive cardiac failure may be the presenting feature, with cardiomegaly and pulmonary congestion.

Cyanosis of the lower extremities is attributable to flow of deoxygenated blood from the pulmonary artery through the patent ductus arteriosus with absence or diminution of the lower limb pulses.

A systolic precordial murmur may be audible.

Electrocardiography may reveal right ventricular or biventricular hypertrophy.

2-D echocardiography defines the interrupted aortic arch and the associated patent ductus arteriosus and ventricular septal defect.

Cardiac catheterization and angiography will define the extent of the aortic arch interruption.

Surgical treatment

As distal perfusion is maintained by the patent ductus, preoperative administration of prostaglandin E_1 is necessary to assure patency of this channel.

Although a two-stage procedure is sometimes indicated, with restoration of aortic continuity and pulmonary artery banding followed later by closure of the ventricular septal defect and pulmonary unbanding, a one-stage repair is preferred whenever possible.

Repair of interrupted aortic arch

A midline sternotomy provides access for extracorporeal circulation, deep hypothermia and circulatory arrest.

The ductus arteriosus, left carotid and left subclavian arteries and descending aorta are mobilized. The ductus is ligated and vascular clamps are placed on the descending aorta and obliquely across the aortic arch and left carotid artery.

The ductal tissue beyond the ligature is excised to prevent narrowing of the subsequent anastomosis. The arch and left carotid artery are incised at the latter's origin and the mobilized descending aorta is anastomosed end-to-side to the incised arch with a continuous posterior suture and interrupted anterior sutures.

If the gap between the transverse arch and the descending aorta is too great, a prosthetic bridging graft can be used.

Bypass is then instituted and the ventricular septal defect closed in standard manner.

Further Reading

Crafoord C., Nylin G. Congenital coarctation of the aorta and its surgical treatment. *J. Thorac. Surg.* 14: 347, 1945.

Gross R. E. Surgical correction for coarctation of the aorta. *Surgery* 18: 673, 1945.

Harlan J. L., Dory D. B., Brandy B., Ehrenhaft J. L. Coarctation of the aorta in infants. *J. Thorac. Cardiovasc. Surg.* 88: 1012, 1984.

Marks P., Marks C. Coarctation of the aorta. In: Marks C. (Ed.), *Surgical management of systemic hypertension.* Futura Publishing Co. Inc. Mt Kisco, New York. 1981.

Waldhausen J. A., Whitman V., Werner J. C., Pierce W. S. Surgical intervention in infants with coarctation of the aorta. *J. Thorac. Cardiovasc. Surg.* 81: 323, 1981.

Chapter 24
Aortic Arch Anomalies

Embryology

The truncus arteriosus commences as a common arterial trunk emerging from the bulbus cordis. During the first 3 weeks of embryonic life, six pairs of aortic arches join the ventral aortic sac and the paired dorsal aortas around the interposed pharynx. The aortas caudal to the paired arches fuse to become an unpaired dorsal descending aorta (Fig. 24.1).

The first and second arches rapidly disappear.

The third arch on each side becomes the common carotid artery.

The fourth arch on the right side becomes the innominate and right subclavian artery.

The fourth arch on the left side becomes the definitive aortic arch, giving off the left subclavian artery and linking up distally with the descending aorta.

The fifth arch disappears.

AORTIC ARCH ANOMALIES WITH VASCULAR RINGS

Clinical Anatomy:

(i). Remnants of aortic arch system

(ii). Dysphagia lusoria: Compression of osephagus and trachea

(iii). Double aortic arch

(iv). Retroesophageal subclavian artery

Fig. 24.1. Clinical anatomy of aortic arch anomalies.

The sixth arch forms the right and left pulmonary arteries after the truncus arteriosus has developed its longitudinal spiral partition to divide off the ascending aorta and pulmonary trunk.

On the left side the sixth arch retains its connection with the dorsal aorta to provide the ductus arteriosus, which normally closes at, or soon after, birth to become the ligamentum arteriosum.

This pattern of development accounts for the fact that the recurrent laryngeal nerve winds round the subclavian artery on the right side and around the aortic arch on the left side — both derived from the fourth arch and explained by the fact that during maturation, the embryo develops an elongated neck while the heart migrates caudally.

A peritracheal and perioesophageal ring develops when both aortic arches persist or when aortic arch branches of anomalous origin occur.

The vascular compression of the trachea and oesophagus (dysphagia lusoria) causes dyspnoea, crowing respiration and dysphagia.

Radiological examination with barium swallow will demonstrate the oesophageal compression (Fig. 24.2) while arteriography will define the nature of the abnormality (Fig. 24.3).

Types

Double aortic arch

The small ventral arch is usually situated to the left or anterior to the main arch. The left arch is best approached through a left 4th interspace thoracotomy, with release of the constricting factor by mobilizing and dividing it between the left carotid and left subclavian arteries. The ligamentum arteriosum or patent ductus must also be divided near its junction with the aortic isthmus, and the aortic arch is mobilized sufficiently to relieve the tracheal compression.

Right aortic arch

The right aortic arch may be associated with a vascular diverticulum that arises from the descending aorta, protruding behind the oesophagus. The ligamentum arteriosum and the left subclavian artery arise from it, with compressive effects. Division of the ligamentum arteriosum is usually curative. Rarely is it necessary to divide the left subclavian artery.

Innominate artery compression
Anomalous origin of the innominate and carotid arteries from the distal left-sided aortic arch will cause tracheal compression. The arch and its anomalous branches will need to be suspended from the anterior chest wall with interrupted pledgeted ticron sutures to alleviate the compression.

Anomalous right subclavian artery
The right subclavian artery arises anomalously from the distal aortic arch and runs to the right behind the oesophagus. The artery should be detached from its anomalous origin and re-implanted in end-to-side fashion to the partially occluded ascending aorta.

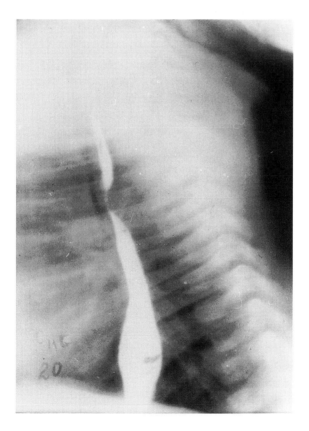

Fig. 24.2. Oesophagogram delineates oesophageal compression by vascular ring.

Pulmonary artery sling

An anomalous origin of the left pulmonary artery from the right pulmonary artery, causes it to pass between the trachea and oesophagus to reach the left lung. Associated abnormalities of the heart and tracheobronchial tree are often present.

Via a midline sternotomy the left pulmonary artery is mobilized from behind the trachea and the ligamentum arteriosum divided. The artery is divided at its origin from the right pulmonary artery and the proximal end ligated. The left pulmonary artery is then anastomosed to the partially occluded main pulmonary artery.

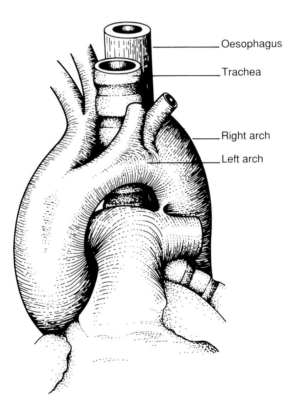

Oesophagus

Trachea

Right arch

Left arch

Fig. 24.3. Double aortic arch.

Further Reading

Edwards J. E. Anomalies of the derivatives of the aortic arch system. *Med. Clin. N. Am.* p. 925, July 1948.

Richardson J. V., Doty D. B., Rossi N. P., Ehrenhaft J. L. Operation for aortic arch anomalies. *Ann. Thorac. Surg.* 3: 426, 1981.

Sade R. M., Rosenthal A., Fellows K., Castaneda A. R. Pulmonary artery sling. *J. Thorac. Cardiovasc. Surg.* 69: 333, 1975.

Chapter 25
Congenital Aortic Stenosis

Congenital aortic stenosis

Obstruction to left ventricular outflow can occur below the valve (infravalvular), at the valve itself (valvular) or above the valve (supravalvular) (Fig. 25.1).

Embryological basis

During the 6th to 9th week of gestation, as truncus arteriosus septation into aorta and pulmonary artery develops, the aortic valves first

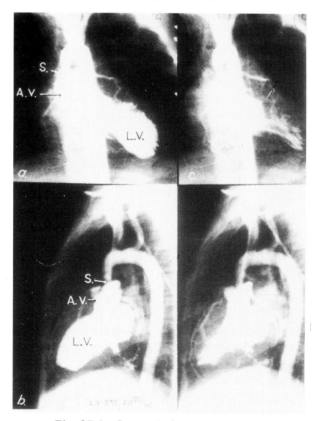

Fig. 25.1. Congenital aortic stenosis.
A Valvular.   B Supravalvular.

appear as three proliferative tubercles within the aortic lumen. The tubercles grow towards the midline while resorption of tissue at the junction of the tubercles and aortic wall gives rise to the three valve sinuses. At this time development of the coronary arteries is completed. Congenital deficiency of the media between the aortic wall and the annulus fibrosus of the aortic valves will predispose to the development of aneurysms of the aortic sinuses of Valsalva.

Valvular stenosis

This is the most common variety and is often associated with a bicuspid valve. It may present in the neonatal period with severe obstruction to left ventricular outflow and ensuing congestive cardiac failure.

More commonly the condition is asymptomatic, being detected at routine clinical examination when a harsh systolic ejection murmur is heard over the second right intercostal space, with radiation into the neck. A palpable thrill may accompany the murmur.

Stenosis of a tricuspid aortic valve is rarely associated with incompetence but bicuspid valve stenosis often demonstrates concomitant regurgitation, with a diastolic murmur audible along the left sternal border.

The development of exertional syncope, arrhythmia and even sudden death are events that should be anticipated by accurate diagnosis and timely remedial treatment.

Radiological examination of the chest

The heart may be normal in size but prominence of the ascending aorta will develop because of the post-stenotic dilatation. Left ventricular hypertrophy and cardiomegaly may occur, with a tight stenosis and high pressure gradient.

Electrocardiography

This may reflect the left ventricular hypertrophy but the development of left ventricular strain with ST depression indicates a high gradient and demands early operative relief of the obstruction.

2-D echocardiography

This will identify the bicuspid nature of the stenosed valve and may define the concentric ventricular hypertrophic thickening.

The echo-dense aortic valve will show restricted motion. This study will also identify the presence of subaortic obstruction or a supravalvular constriction.

Cardiac catheterization

This will permit measurement of the pressure gradient across the obstruction. A systolic gradient greater than 50 mmHg in valvular stenosis provides a strong indication for valvotomy. Surgical repair may be indicated with a lower gradient in subvalvular or supravalvular obstruction, as deformation of the aortic valve may cause aortic incompetence.

Angiography will identify the exact type of obstruction and the presence of associated valve incompetence.

Delineation of the coronary arteries and the demonstration of hypoplasia of the sinuses of Valsalva may provide important pre-operative information.

Surgical management

A midline sternotomy, cardiopulmonary bypass and cardioplegic arrest with left ventricular venting permits all subsequent manoeuvres in all forms of left ventricular outflow tract obstruction.

An oblique aortotomy extending into the non-coronary cusp will expose the valvular stenosis. There is usually a bicuspid valve with both commissures fused and a raphe indicating the location of the vestigial commissure. The conjoined leaflet is the unicusp and the opening between the unicusp and the other single cusp is slit-like with an eccentric orifice.

A valvotomy is performed, incising the commissures in the midline and dilating the orifice with Hegar dilators. Finger palpation of the subaortic region to exclude an association subvalvular membrane is followed by closure of the aortotomy incision with pledgeted 4-0 prolene sutures, reinforced by a second row of sutures.

Subvalvular stenosis

Hypertrophic idiopathic subaortic stenosis (HISS)

This is due to inappropriately hypertrophied heart muscle, which contracts during systole. The aortic valve is seen to be normal at echocardiographic examination.

Discrete subvalvular membranous stenosis
A fibrous ring with a narrowed central orifice is situated just below the normal aortic valves. Associated aortic insufficiency is often present.

Treatment: An aortotomy is fashioned and the valve leaflets are retracted. The underlying diaphragm or membrane is exposed and carefully dissected from the left ventricular outflow tract and separated from the underlying myocardium. Careful dissection in the mitral valve region will peel the fibrotic tissue off the adjacent structures. The separation of the membrane from the ventricular septum should be done with care so as not to perforate it or injure the conduction system. The normal aortic leaflets must not be damaged.

Morrow operation: In hypertrophic idiopathic subaortic stenosis the asymmetric hypertrophy of the septum in the left ventricular outflow tract results in systolic anterior motion of the ventral leaflet of the mitral valve.

The aortic leaflets are retracted through an aortotomy, so that the bulging ventricular septum can be visualized.

The muscle bar just to the right of centre of the right coronary cusp is identified and a 2 cm deep incision is made into the ventricular muscle. A second incision is made 12 mm to the left of the first incision. The intervening wedge of muscle is excised by connecting incisions. After lavage of the left ventricle to remove any debris, the aortotomy is closed.

Supravalvular stenosis
This is rare and is due to a narrowing of a long segment of the aorta above the normal aortic valves. The coronary arteries are greatly dilated in this condition, which is often familial. It may be associated with infantile hypercalcaemia and may be part of William's syndrome: elfin facies, mental retardation with supravalvular stenoses of aorta and pulmonary artery.

Treatment
A vertical aortotomy across the constricted area extends into the non-coronary sinus. The internal shelf is excised and the lumen enlarged with a preclotted dacron patch or a patch of glutaraldehyde-treated

pericardium, sutured into place with 5-0 prolene sutures. Pledgeted mattress sutures are used at the cusp area.

Sinus of Valsalva aneurysms and fistulae

Congenital deficiency of the media between the aortic wall and the annulus fibrosus of the aortic valves predisposes to aneurysm formation at the aortic sinuses.

Rarely such aneurysms may be luetic or mycotic in origin. The aneurysms project into the adjacent cardiac chambers:

1   Right coronary sinus aneurysm into right ventricle
2   Non-coronary sinus aneurysm into right atrium
3   Left coronary sinus aneurysm into left atrium or pericardium.

Unruptured aneurysms are asymptomatic as there are no disturbances of cardiac function.

Rupture of the aneurysm creates a shunt between the aorta and the appropriate cardiac chamber, with sudden onset of chest pain followed by congestive cardiac failure and the presence of an audible continuous precordial murmur.

Radiologically the chest is normal until the aneurysm ruptures, when cardiomegaly develops rapidly.

Electrocardiography rapidly reveals the development of bi-ventricular hypertrophy and arrhythmias.

2-D echocardiography identifies the aortic root aneurysm while Doppler studies will demonstrate blood flow from the aorta through the fistula to the appropriate cardiac chamber.

Cardiac catheterization reveals increased oxygen saturation in the corresponding heart chamber. Aortography outlines the fistulous shunt.

An accompanying ventricular septal defect is occasionally revealed, requiring placement of a patch during the operative procedure.

Treatment

A midline sternotomy and cardiopulmonary bypass are utilized. The aortic root is opened and cardioplegia solution perfused directly into the coronary ostia.

The aneurysm and fistula are exposed and probed. Occasionally a "wind-sock" can be withdrawn into the aortic root and excised (Fig. 25.2). The defect is then closed with a dacron patch using interrupted sutures so as not to distort the aortic leaflets.

If a prosthetic aortic valve replacement is necessary for concomitant valve disease, the sinus defect is incorporated into the sutures used to attach the valve prosthesis, its sewing ring being used to buttress the repairs.

Further Reading

Campbell M. The natural history of congenital aortic stenosis. *Br. Heart J.* 30: 514, 1968.

Kirklin J. W., Barratt-Boyes B. G. Congenital aortic stenosis. In: Kirklin J. W., Barratt-Boyes B. G. (Eds), *Cardiac surgery.* John Wiley and Sons. New York. 1986.

Meyer J., Wukasch D. C., Hallman G. L., Cooley D. A. Aneurysm and fistula of the sinus of Valsalva: Clinical considerations and surgical treatment in 45 patients. *Ann. Thorac. Surg.* 19: 170, 1975.

Morrow A. G. Hypertrophic subaortic stenosis: Operative methods utilized to relieve left ventricular outflow obstruction. *J. Thorac. Cardiovasc. Surg.* 76: 403, 1978.

Oldham H. N. Jr. Congenital aortic stenosis. In: Sabiston D. C. (Ed.), *Textbook of surgery: The biological basis of modern surgical practice.* 13th ed. W. B. Saunders Co. Philadelphia. 1986.

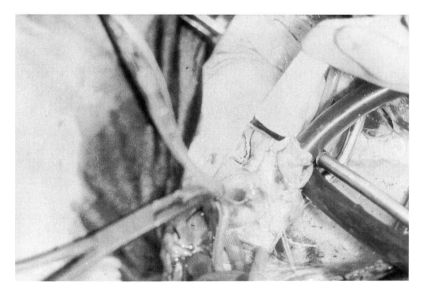

Fig. 25.2. Sinus of Valsalva aneurysm creating a "wind-sock" that can be excised.

Chapter 26
Pulmonary Stenosis and Right Ventricular
Outflow Tract Obstruction

Pulmonary stenosis is a common form of congenital heart disease representing 10% of all types of congenital cardiac disorder.

It may be valvular, infundibular or combined valvular and infundibular stenosis, either existing alone or in association with:

1 Atrial septal defect
2 Ventricular septal defect with a normal aortic root
3 Ventricular septal defect with a dextroposed aorta: Fallot's Tetralogy.

Supravalvular pulmonary stenosis may occur.

Types of pulmonary stenosis
Valvular
Failure of normal development of the three pulmonary valve leaflets leads to the valvular form of pulmonary stenosis, with thickening and partial or total fusion at their commissures. This results in a funnel-shaped domed valve with a central small orifice. Occasionally only two leaflets develop, with fusion at their common commissures.

Infundibular
Failure of normal resorption of tissue in the subjacent bulbus cordis results in an area of infundibular hypertrophy, which causes the less common variety of infundibular pulmonary stenosis.

Abnormal bands of muscle
Abnormal bands of muscle may be deposited within the body of the right ventricle causing varying degrees of right outflow tract obstruction.

Established valvular pulmonary stenosis may cause delayed development or infundibular hypertrophy and stenosis.

Supravalvular pulmonary artery stenosis
At about the 8th week of gestation, the pulmonary valve develops concomitantly with the truncus arteriosus. Three tubercles within

186

the lumen of the primitive pulmonary artery trunk grow intra-
luminally and become thinned by resorption of tissue.

The right ventricular infundibulum develops from the proximal
portion of the bulbus cordis. At this time differentiation of the
aortic arch system occurs, with the sixth arch becoming the distal
portion of the pulmonary trunk. The pulmonary trunk connects
distally with the smaller pulmonary arteries derived from the
pulmonary artery. At these sites of embryological junction various
forms of supravalvular pulmonary stenosis may develop:

1 Type I: single constriction of main trunk or of the right or left
   pulmonary artery
2 Type II: stenosis at the bifurcation of the main pulmonary trunk
3 Type III: multiple peripheral stenoses
4 Type IV: combination of Types I and III.

Haemodynamic effects

The systolic pulmonary artery and right ventricular pressure is
increased as the right ventricle has to pump against the obstruction,
but the diastolic pressure remains unchanged.

Circulation to the lungs is diminished while the right ventricle
and right atrium undergo hypertrophy. There is reduced pulmonary
venous return, with reduction in left ventricular outflow.

In valvular stenosis there is marked post-stenotic dilatation of
the main pulmonary artery which is demonstrable on chest X-ray
(Fig. 26.1) and pulmonary arteriography.

If the obstruction is infundibular in location, dissipation of the
right ventricular force through the elongated obstructed area
eliminates the post-stenotic effect and there is no pulmonary artery
dilatation.

Radiological examination of the chest will reveal the diminished
vascularity of the lung fields and the right ventricular hypertrophy,
with an upturned apex in the postero-anterior view and an anterior
bulge of the cardiac shadow in the left lateral view.

Electrocardiography demonstrates features of right ventricular
hypertrophy with right axis deviation in both forms of pulmonary
stenosis. There is usually good correlation between the degree of
right ventricular hypertrophy and the degree of pulmonary stenosis.

Clinical features

1 The patient is asymptomatic. Valvular pulmonary stenosis is more common in males and the abnormality is detected during a routine medical examination, with a palpable thrill in the second left intercostal space and a systolic ejection murmur at the pulmonic area, radiating to the back.

   The ejection click is audible in valvular but not in infundibular stenosis. The second sound may be split, with a diminished pulmonic component.

   With a pronounced valvular pulmonary stenosis, hypertrophy of the right ventricle and its outflow tract may cause a

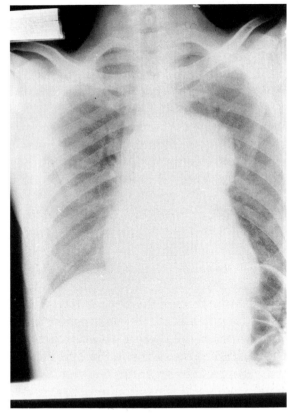

Fig. 26.1. Congential pulmonary valve stenosis with post-stenotic dilatation demonstrated radiologically.

superimposed secondary infundibular stenosis.

2 The patient may develop fatigue and shortness of breath on exertion due to diminished right ventricular outflow.

3 In infancy acute heart failure may develop suddenly at about 6 months of age due to restriction of right ventricular output. There is an increase in end-diastolic pressure, with tricuspid insufficiency and an increase in right atrial pressure.

Dilatation of the right atrium with incompetence of the foramen ovale leads to a right-to-left shunt. The development of cyanosis alongside the existent congestive heart failure may require an immediate life-saving operation (Fig. 26.2).

Neonatal right heart failure due to pulmonary stenosis may

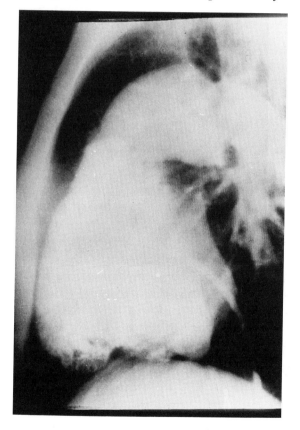

Fig. 26.2. Pulmonary arteriography delineates valvular stenosis.

cause difficulty in differentiating it from pulmonary atresia.

Echocardiography will demonstrate the level and severity of pulmonary stenosis.

Cardiac catheterization can confirm the clinical diagnosis. Based on right ventricular and pulmonary artery pressures, the degree of stenotic severity and pressure gradient can be established.

Angiocardiography will demonstrate the stenotic architecture and will define any associated cardiac anomalies.

Noonan syndrome
Pulmonary valvular dysplasia causing pulmonary stenosis is associated with small stature, hypertelorism, mild mental retardation and skeletal abnormalities as well as ptosis and cryptorchidism.

Surgical management
Critical pulmonary stenosis in infancy requires an emergency transventricular pulmonary valvotomy.

The heart is exposed via a median sternotomy. A mattress suture of pledgeted 4–0 prolene is placed in the right ventricular outflow tract. A 5 mm Brock knife is advanced into the pulmonary artery through a stab wound, and the stenosed valve is incised. A rongeur is then used to excise the annular valve tissue. The myocardial mattress suture is tied and the mediastinum is closed.

In children and adults, cardiopulmonary bypass with cardioplegic arrest is established via a midline sternotomy. The pulmonary artery is opened vertically and the dome-shaped valve exposed.

The three commissures are incised well back into the annulus, but if the valve is bicuspid both commissures are incised, staying in the centre of the fused commissure to avoid valvular insufficiency and incompetence.

Balloon valvuloplasty
Since the first successful balloon dilatation of the stenosed pulmonary valve in 1982, the procedure is now recommended in all cases of congenital pulmonary valve stenosis except in patients with dysplastic valves, invalidating the need for open heart procedures.

The procedure is performed by cardiologists using right heart catheterization techniques, utilizing two balloon catheters introduced via a femoral vein. It is indicated in patients with a gradient of 50 mmHg or greater across the valve, or in patients with a lesser gradient if right ventricular hypertrophy is present.

Rapid inflation of the properly placed balloon catheters to 3–4 atmospheres pressure, using dilute contrast material, followed by rapid deflation, usually reduces the gradient to less than 20 mmHg.

Balloon valvuloplasty has also been utilized in aortic stenosis, mitral stenosis and re-coarctation of the aorta.

Further Reading

Anderson I.M., Nouri-Moghaddam S. Severe pulmonary stenosis in infancy and early childhood. *Thorax* 24: 312, 1969.

Coles J.G., Freedom R.M., Olley P.M. *et al.* Surgical management of critical pulmonary stenosis in the neonate. *Ann. Thorac. Surg.* 38: 485, 1984.

Danilowicz D., Hoffman J.I.E., Rudolph A.M. Serial studies of pulmonary stenosis in infancy and childhood. *Br. Heart J.* 37: 808, 1975.

McKay R.G. Balloon valvuloplasty for treating pulmonic, mitral and aortic valve stenoses. *Am. J. Cardiol.* 61: 1026, 1988.

Chapter 27
Tetralogy of Fallot

Fallot's tetralogy is the most common form of congenital cyanotic heart disease. The anomaly comprises:

1 A high large membranous interventricular septal defect
2 Right ventricular outflow tract obstruction
3 Dextroposition of the aorta which over-rides the ventricular septum
4 Right ventricular hypertrophy.

The degree of right ventricular outflow tract obstruction may range from slight pulmonary stenosis to complete atresia. Although infundibular stenosis is most commonly present, a combination of valvular and infundibular stenosis may occur.

The septal defect is situated in the membranous or subaortic part of the interventricular septum.

The over-riding of the aorta is attributable to an abnormality of the aortic root, with the aorta malaligned in relation to the left ventricular outflow tract. By being displaced to the right, or dextroposed, the aorta overlies or over-rides the interventricular septum from which it is separated by the high defect (Fig. 27.1).

Right ventricle hypertrophy represents the haemodynamic response to the other three abnormalities.

The commonest associated congenital anomalies are:

1 A right sided aortic arch
2 Persistent left superior vena cava.

Embryological anatomy
Asymmetric septation of the truncus arteriosus results in inequality in the size of the two great vessels. This asymmetry creates unavailability of that portion of the membranous septum that would normally close the atrioventricular area, resulting in a large ventricular septal defect.

Infundibular stenosis develops because of an excessive amount of tissue in the infundibular area as a result of the asymmetry.

There is a consistent hypertrophy of the crista supraventricularis, hypoplasia of the pulmonary valve annulus with pulmonary valvular stenosis, and a subcristal defect that equals the size of the aortic lumen.

The crista supraventricularis is a muscular ridge located below the pulmonary valves and separates the infundibulum from the rest of the right ventricular cavity.

Haemodynamics

There is diminished blood flow to the lungs, with unsaturated blood flowing across the ventricular septal defect from right to left causing central cyanosis. The severity of the effects depends on the degree of pulmonary stenosis. The more severe the right outflow

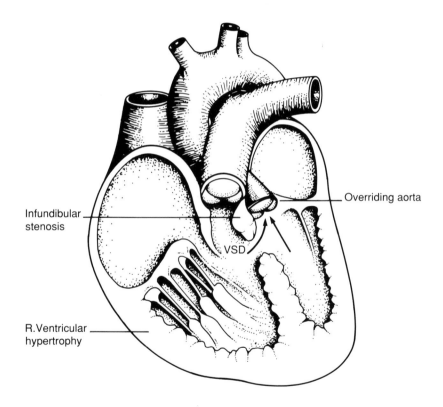

Infundibular stenosis

Overriding aorta

VSD

R.Ventricular hypertrophy

Fig. 27.1. Fallot's tetralogy.

tract obstruction the earlier the clinical presentation and the more severe the cyanosis.

It is unusual for the condition to be obvious at birth, usually taking time to develop with deepening cyanosis as the child grows.

Severe cyanotic episodes may occur intermittently with "spells" due to spasm of the infundibular outflow tract.

Such hypoxic spells may cause unconsciousness and respond well to treatment with beta-blockers such as propranolol, which relieves infundibular spasm.

Compensatory responses to these haemodynamic changes may develop:

1 *Polycythemia*: This response to the anoxia may aggravate the level of cyanosis.
2 *Delayed closure of patent ductus arteriosus*: By deviating blood from the aorta to the pulmonary artery, improved oxygenation is fostered temporarily as the ductus usually closes by 1 year of age.
3 *Collateral circulation between systemic and pulmonary arterial systems*: Bronchial, mediastinal, oesophageal, internal mammary and pericardial arteries permit flow from the aortic to the pulmonary artery system for oxygenation.

Clinical features

Although the occasional patient may survive to middle age, most die before entering the second decade. Cyanosis, clubbing of fingers and toes and polycythaemia develop in older babies and children.

There is marked dyspnoea on exertion and the child prefers to squat, thereby increasing peripheral arterial resistance and favourably influencing pulmonary blood flow. Failure to thrive and stunted growth are noticeable.

The heart is not enlarged and a loud precordial systolic murmur is present, maximally audible over the left second and third interspaces, and attributable to pulmonary stenosis.

Radiographic chest examination confirms a normal sized heart with a "boot-shaped" configuration – *coeur en sabot* – due to the hypertrophied right ventricle displacing the left ventricle up and to the left. The narrow waist is due to hypoplasia of the pulmonary artery. Hilar oligaemia is attributable to the reduced pulmonary blood flow.

Electrocardiography reflects right ventricular hypertrophy and strain as well as right atrial hypertrophy.

2-D echocardiography will demonstrate the characteristic over-riding of the aorta and will reflect the size of the pulmonary arteries. These features can also be defined by radioactive scanning (Fig. 27.2).

Cardiac catheterization and angiography will define the anatomy of the right ventricular outflow tract, the pulmonary artery size and the high-lying ventricular septal defect with simultaneous opacification of the aorta and pulmonary artery.

Complications of tetralogy may provide confusing clinical manifestations:

1 Subacute bacterial endocarditis
2 Cardiac failure is an uncommon manifestation as the septal defect provides a safety valve for the elevated right ventricular pressure
3 Cerebral thrombosis with hemiplegia, due to the polycythaemia
4 Brain abscess due to a paradoxical infected embolus from a peripheral vein passing through the ventricular septal defect. Secondary infection of a cerebral infarct may complicate cerebral thrombosis.

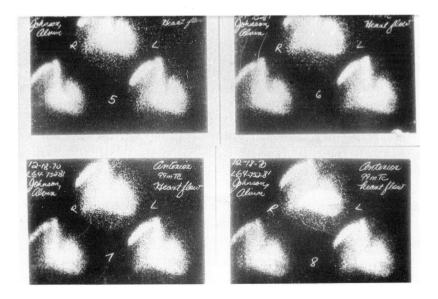

Fig. 27.2. Radioactive scan defines the over-riding aorta and pulmonary stenosis.

Surgical management

Complete atresia of the pulmonary valve usually requires operative intervention shortly after birth, as effective pulmonary blood flow will cease with closure of the ductus arteriosus.

If operative intervention is necessary in the early months of life, a systemic–pulmonary shunt is indicated for palliation but whenever possible operative intervention should be delayed so that total correction can be carried out when the child is older. At the time of total correction, a previously fashioned shunt will need to be obliterated.

Blalock–Taussig anastomosis

Classically the shunt is constructed on the side opposite to the aortic arch, i.e. left arch: right-sided anastomosis.

A 4th interspace right posterolateral thoracotomy provides good access. After insertion of the rib-spreader the lung is retracted down and posteriorly. The pleura over the right pulmonary artery is incised and the artery dissected out. The pulmonary vein draining the upper lobe lies anterior and inferior to the artery. Silk ties are placed around the pulmonary artery branches for distal control.

The mediastinal pleura posterior to the superior vena cava is incised and the azygos vein is doubly ligated and divided. The subclavian artery is mobilized above and below the vagus and its recurrent laryngeal nerve. The innominate and common carotid arteries are mobilized and occlusion ties placed around them.

The subclavian artery is ligated above the origin of the vertebral artery, which is also ligated to prevent a subsequent "steal syndrome". The subclavian artery is occluded with a vascular clamp proximal to the recurrent laryngeal nerve and divided proximal to its point of ligation. It is then turned down below the nerve to the pulmonary artery.

The pulmonary artery is occluded proximally with a vascular clamp, its distal branches occluded and a 4 mm longitudinal incision made on the superior aspect of the pulmonary artery.

An end-to-side anastomosis is fashioned using a posterior continuous everting suture of 6-0 prolene, fixed at each end to an anchoring stitch. The anterior anastomotic line utilizes 6-0 prolene interrupted sutures.

All occlusive ties are loosened, clamps removed and a continuous thrill palpated at the junction of the systemic–pulmonary anastomosis.

The chest is closed with a thoracotomy drainage tube, which is removed 24 hours later.

Great Ormond Street variation
This has become the current procedure of choice. A direct shunt of Gore-tex or impra avoids sacrifice of the subclavian artery flow but is liable to thrombosis. The procedure is generally performed on the left side with a 4–5 mm interposition graft between the left subclavian and left pulmonary arteries and is appropriate in infants utilizing proximal and distal end-to-side anastomoses.

Waterston anastomosis
This procedure has a place in infants with a very small pulmonary artery, and permits anastomosis between the ascending aorta and the right pulmonary artery, as an intrapericardial aortopulmonary anastomosis.

Access is via a right anterior 4th interspace thoracotomy. The pericardium is opened anterior to the right phrenic nerve.

The ascending aorta is retracted leftward and the pulmonary artery exposed between the aorta and the superior vena cava to its right. The pulmonary artery is freed and heavy silk controlling sutures placed around its two branches. A vascular clamp is placed proximally with its posterior blade behind the right pulmonary artery and the anterior blade occluding the adjacent segment of aorta. Parallel 3 mm incisions in the aorta and pulmonary artery are made and interrupted 6-0 prolene sutures create an anastomosis between the two. After removal of the occluding distal pulmonary ties and the vascular clamp, the chest is closed.

At the time of subsequent total correction, this shunt can be closed by opening the aortic root and obliterating the anastomosis by suture from within.

Potts' aortopulmonary anastomosis
Because of the difficulty in closing this shunt at the time of total repair, this procedure is rarely used in tetralogy of Fallot.

Through a left 4th interspace posterolateral thoracotomy, the left lung is depressed and the mediastinal pleura incised over the aorta. The anterior surface of the aorta is cleared and the left main pulmonary artery mobilized. It is controlled by encircling silk sutures proximally and its branches distally. The aorta is partially occluded by a curved vascular clamp and, after approximating the left pulmonary artery and the aorta, 4 mm incisions are made in both vessels; an anastomosis is fashioned with 5-0 continuous prolene suture.

Total correction of tetralogy of Fallot

It is the general consensus that during and after the first year of life, immediate total correction should be done whenever possible, thereby avoiding the psychological effects and the morbidity and mortality of two operations, or the need to undo the palliative procedure, which may induce problems of its own.

A midline sternotomy, cardiopulmonary bypass with hypothermia and cardioplegic arrest with venting of the left ventricle set the stage for the repair.

An incision over the right ventricular outflow tract extends from the pulmonary annulus to a point below the crista supraventricularis. Any coronary artery branches should be avoided.

After assessment of the pathological anatomy, the infundibular resection is accomplished with excision of any parietal or septal bands.

The ventricular septal defect is closed with a dacron patch: a concomitant atrial septal defect or foramen ovale is searched for in the right atrium and, if present, closed.

The pulmonary valve is opened through an incision in the pulmonary artery: the dome-shaped valve is exposed and the commissures carefully incised well back into the annulus. The annulus is calibrated with Hegar dilators after completion of the pulmonary valvotomy. If calibration indicates that the annulus needs to be enlarged then an incision is carried across the annulus in the commissures between two valve cusps to avoid subsequent regurgitation.

The entire outflow tract, including the infundibulum, annulus and, if necessary, main pulmonary artery is enlarged by closing it with a pericardial patch, which is sutured in position with 4-0 prolene.

Right ventricular to pulmonary artery conduit

The association of pulmonary atresia and ventricular septal defect will require placement of an external conduit after patch closure of the ventricular septal defect. Under these circumstances, total correction is delayed until the child is about 6 years of age, so that an appropriate-sized conduit can be used.

A preliminary systemic–pulmonary shunt will be necessary and will be closed at the time of total correction.

The pulmonary artery and right ventricle are incised via a midline sternotomy and cardiopulmonary bypass, and after patch closure of the ventricular septal defect a 22 mm valved conduit is sutured to the pulmonary artery with the valve as close as possible to the artery. The conduit is tailored proximally for continuous 3-0 prolene suture to the ventriculotomy.

Further Reading

Blalock A., Taussig H. B. The surgical treatment of malformation of the heart in which there is pulmonary stenosis or pulmonary atresia. *J.A.M.A.* 128: 189, 1945.

Kirklin J. W., Karp R. B. *The tetralogy of Fallot from a surgical viewpoint.* W. B. Saunders Co. Philadelphia. 1970.

Potts W. J., Smith S., Gibson S. Anastomosis of the aorta to a pulmonary artery for certain types of congenital heart disease. *J.A.M.A.* 132: 629, 1946.

Sabiston D. C. Jr. The tetralogy of Fallot. In: Sabiston D. C. Jr (Ed.), *Textbook of surgery.* 13th edition. W. B. Saunders Co. Philadelphia. 1986.

Waterston D. J. Treatment of Fallot's tetralogy in children under 1 year of age. *Rozhl. Chir.* 41: 181, 1962.

Chapter 28
Disorders of the Tricuspid Valve

Tricuspid atresia

In tricuspid atresia there is no vestige of valvular tissue, the small thickened non-perforated membrane preventing any communication between the right atrium and the right ventricle. There is always an associated atrial septal defect or a patent foramen ovale. The right ventricle is small, rudimentary and filled with blood clot.

Embryological basis

The right atrioventricular or tricuspid valve is normally formed by a blending of the anterior and posterior endocardial cushions with a segment of interventricular septum and ventricular muscle. The process is completed by about the fifth week of gestation, at which time the associated papillary muscles and chordae tendinae develop from fine sculpturing of the ventricular muscle.

Disruption in the balance between proliferation and resorbtion adversely affects the valve leaflet formation, with atresia as the end result.

Associated anomalies

1 Normally related great vessels:
   a) No ventricular septal defect or pulmonary stenosis
   b) Small VSD and pulmonary stenosis
   c) Large VSD without pulmonary stenosis.
2 Transposition of great vessels:
   a) VSD and pulmonary atresia
   b) VSD and pulmonary stenosis
   c) VSD without pulmonary stenosis.

Clinical features

Cyanosis: The central cyanosis is usually severe from birth. This is followed by polycythaemia and clubbing of the fingers and toes.

Shortness of breath on exertion, fatigue, failure to thrive and poor physical development are common symptoms.

Congestive cardiac failure, thrombotic phenomena and death in infancy are inevitable if the condition is uncorrected.

Auscultation reveals a single first sound, single second sound and absence of a murmur. If a murmur is present it will be due to an associated ventricular septal defect or pulmonary stenosis.

Haemodynamics

Blood from the right atrium cannot reach the right ventricle, flowing instead into the left atrium via an atrial septal defect or patent foramen ovale. It then passes to the left ventricle and through the aorta to the systemic circulation.

Blood flow to the lungs is possible:

1 Via a patent ductus
2 Via a ventricular septal defect into the rudimentary right ventricle and thence into the pulmonary artery.

Radiological examination

Cardiomegaly is due to a large right atrium with a large left ventricle. The pulmonary vascular markings are diminished with diminution in size or absence of the pulmonary conus.

Electrocardiography will show left ventricular hypertrophy and strain. Tall P waves in leads II, V1 and V2 reflect right atrial hypertrophy.

Echocardiography demonstrates absence of the tricuspid valve and hypoplasia of the right ventricle. Any associated anomalies will be defined.

Cardiac catheterization will confirm the diagnosis of tricuspid atresia, with angiographic demonstration of flow through the atrial septal defect to the left atrium and then to the left ventricle.

An assessment of pulmonary to systemic blood flow is made and the degree of right ventricular outflow tract obstruction and status of the pulmonary arteries are defined.

Surgical treatment

Palliative surgery

This is appropriate in the first two years of life.

1 Blalock systemic–pulmonary type shunt
2 Glenn shunt: an anastomosis between the superior vena cava and the pulmonary artery. Rarely done as recurrence of cyanosis occurs due to arteriovenous malformations. The right

pulmonary artery is divided medial to the superior vena cava.
An intracaval catheter is placed via a right atriotomy and tape
occlusion above and below permits continued caval flow to the
right atrium. An oval segment of SVC is excised and an end-to-
side pulmonary–caval anastomosis created.

Fontan procedure
Designed so as to permit flow of blood from the right atrium to the
pulmonary artery. A low pulmonary vascular resistance and a
large pulmonary artery are essential for a successful performance
of this procedure.

If the right ventricle is present, even if small, and there is an
adequate pulmonary annulus then a right atrium to right ventricle
connection is created.

If there is no right ventricle then the atrium must be connected
to the pulmonary artery, either with or without a conduit.

Right atrium to right ventricle connection
The operation is ideally performed when the child is 8–10 years of
age. Via a midline sternotomy, cardiopulmonary bypass, moderate
hypothermia and cardioplegic arrest, the right ventricle is incised
and a patch applied to the ventricular septal defect if present.
1 The right atrial appendage is amputated and a patch placed
   over a patent foramen ovale or atrial septal defect. A woven
   fabric conduit (16–20 mm diameter) is then fashioned from
   right atrium to right ventricle. Only if there is raised pulmonary
   arterial pressure or a satisfactory pulmonary valve is absent,
   need a valved conduit be used.
2 *Bjork's technique*: Creation of a flap of right atrium permits
   formation of a posterior pedicled communication with the
   ventricular incision. A pericardial or dacron patch is then sutured
   in place to provide the anterior connection between right atrium
   and right ventricle, providing a conduit large enough to accom-
   modate the entire venous return.

Right atrium to pulmonary artery
1 *Without a conduit*: In cases where there is transposition of the
   great vessels with the pulmonary artery to the right of the aorta,

after patching an associated atrial septal defect, a direct suture anastomosis is fashioned between the right atrial appendage and the main pulmonary artery.

2 *With a conduit*: In normally aligned great vessels, the atrium is connected to the pulmonary artery with a 20 mm non-valved dacron conduit, after closing the ASD.

In both techniques the pulmonary artery is transected and its proximal end closed with a pericardial patch. The atrio-pulmonary connection is then fashioned to the distal opening of the transected artery.

Ebstein's anomaly

The normal development of the tricuspid valve may be disrupted, with displacement of the tricuspid annulus downwards into the right ventricle.

Part of the normal right ventricle becomes incorporated into the right atrium, with foreshortening of its chordae tendinae.

The right atrium is large, the right ventricle is small and the tricuspid valve potentially or actually deformed and incompetent.

Right bundle branch block, either partial or complete, is frequent electrocardiographically, because of disruption of the right-sided bundle of His as it courses adjacent to the tricuspid annulus. Anomalous conduction pathways across the tricuspid annulus may result in the Wolff–Parkinson–White syndrome.

Haemodynamics

The course of the circulation is normal, but as the pressure in the right atrium is increased blood is shunted through the atrial septal defect from right to left. The increased right atrial pressure is due to:

1 Impaired filling of the right ventricle due to obstructive effects of the deformed valve
2 Cardiac failure due to tricuspid incompetence.

Clinical features

1 Heart failure develops due to the impaired filling of the right ventricle or the incompetent tricuspid valve, with distended neck veins, hepatomegaly and ascites.

2   Central cyanosis becomes progressively more severe as the right
    atrial pressure increases.
3   Arrhythmias: episodes of paroxysmal tachycardia.
4   Heart sounds: a holosystolic murmur of tricuspid incompetence
    is audible at the lower end of the sternum. There is a widely
    split second sound. Triple or quadruple rhythm occurs due to
    extra heart sounds.

Radiological examination

There is gross cardiomegaly due to the enlarged right atrium.
There is diminished vascularity of the lung fields.

Electrocardiography

Tall P waves reflect right atrial hypertrophy with right bundle
branch block. The features of Wolff–Parkinson–White syndrome
are manifest in 25% of cases. Episodes of paroxysmal tachycardia
and first degree heart block may be observed.

2-D echocardiography will delineate the position of the abnormal
tricuspid valve and the atrial septal defect.

Cardiac catheterization reveals elevated right atrial pressure
and the presence of an atrial septal defect. Arteriography will
outline the atrialized segment of the right ventricle.

Surgical treatment

A midline sternotomy permits cardiopulmonary bypass, hypothermia and cardioplegic arrest. The right atrium is opened and
the tricuspid leaflets are seen to be thickened, shortened and
adherent to the ventricular wall. The large billowy anterior leaflet
is reattached in its normal position at the annulus with interrupted
pledgeted mattress sutures which imbricate the atrialized portion
of the right ventricle. Competence of the valve is assured with
several plicating sutures of the anterior commissure.

The atrial septal defect is closed with a pericardial patch. An ellipse
of right atrium is excised to make it smaller and the atrium is closed.

If the tricuspid valve cannot be reconstructed then it should be
excised and replaced by a prosthetic valve.

WPW syndrome

If present, accessory conduction fibres are interrupted to eliminate
tachyarrhythmias.

Fontan procedure

This operation may be indicated in patients with a grossly deformed right ventricle. The atrial septal defect is closed with a patch and the right atrium is anastomosed to the pulmonary artery.

Further Reading

Barnard C. N., Schrire V. Surgical correction of Ebstein's malformation with a prosthetic tricuspid valve. *Surgery* 54: 302, 1963.

Bjork V. O., Olin C. L., Bjarke B. B., Thoren C. A. Right atrial–right ventricular anastomosis for correction of tricuspid atresia. *J. Thorac. Cardiovasc. Surg.* 77: 452, 1979.

Fontan F., Baudet E. Surgical repair of tricuspid atresia. *Thorax* 26: 240, 1971.

Fontan F., De Ville C., Quaegebeur J. *et al.* Repair of tricuspid atresia in 100 patients. *J. Thorac. Cardiovasc. Surg.* 85: 647, 1983.

Mathur M., Glenn W. W. L. Long-term evaluation of cava–pulmonary artery anastomosis. *Surgery* 74: 899, 1973.

Silver M. A., Cohen S. R., McIntosh C. L. *et al.* Late clinical and haemodynamic results after either tricuspid valve replacement or annuloplasty for Ebstein's anomaly of the tricuspid valve. *Am. J. Cardiol.* 54: 627, 1984.

Vlad P. Tricuspid atresia. In: Keith J. D., Rowe R. D., Vlad P. (Eds), *Heart disease in infancy and childhood.* Macmillan. New York. 1978.

Chapter 29
Transposition of the Great Arteries

Embryological anatomy

Between the 3rd and 4th weeks of intrauterine life, the truncus arteriosus is divided by a spiral downgrowth of the truncoconal ridges so that normally the left ventricle empties into the aorta and the right ventricle into the pulmonary artery.

If there is disruption of this normal septation, the septum may grow straight downwards so that the aorta arises from the right ventricle and the pulmonary artery from the left ventricle.

The aortic root comes to lie to the right of the pulmonary artery in the 'D' (dextro) position and is also superior and anterior to it. The pulmonary artery origin is then posterior, inferior and to the left of the aortic root. If the aorta is to the left of the pulmonary root, the condition is defined as "L" (laevo) transposition.

Simple transposition

If the ventricular septum is intact, then the condition is defined as a simple transposition (Fig. 29.1). Communication between right and left circulations occurs through either a patent foramen ovale or a patent ductus arteriosus.

Complex transpositions

There are associated anomalies such as ventricular septal defects or pulmonary outflow tract stenosis.

Cordancy

Transposition can also be categorized as cordant or discordant.
1 *Atrial*: The atrioventricular relationship is concordant if right atrium blood flows to right ventricle and discordant if right atrium empties directly into left ventricle.
2 *Ventricular discordance* is the transposition of the great arteries.

Haemodynamics

Blood from the right ventricle flows into the aorta and from the left ventricle into the pulmonary artery. This situation is incompatible with the infant's survival unless a communication exists between the systemic and pulmonary circulations in simple transposition via:

1   A patent ductus flow from pulmonary artery to aorta
2   Atrial septal defect flow from left to right atrium.

In complex transposition unsaturated blood returns from right atrium to right ventricle and then to left ventricle through the ventricular septal defect, and thence to the pulmonary circulation.

Clinical features

Central cyanosis becomes apparent within a few days of birth and may fluctuate as the ductus arteriosus opens and closes. The patency of the ductus should be maintained for as long as possible with

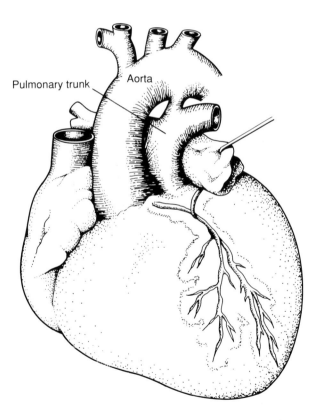

Pulmonary trunk   Aorta

Fig. 29.1. Simple transposition of great vessels.

prostaglandin therapy. The child is usually well developed but signs of congestive failure may develop.

Polycythaemia and clubbing of fingers and toes will occur.

Cardiomegaly develops with right ventricular hypertrophy, and sometimes left ventricular enlargement too, providing a diffuse left parasternal impulse.

Murmurs are usually absent with only a single heart sound audible. Murmurs due to associated shunts may, however, be present.

Progressive deterioration with cyanosis, shortness of breath, hypoxia and acidosis results in death of most untreated infants within 6 months.

Radiological examination

Cardiomegaly is marked, involving both ventricles but more so the right ventricle, providing an "egg-shaped" cardiac silhouette. The plethoric, hyperaemic lung fields in a cyanotic infant are highly characteristic and make the diagnosis of transposition very likely.

Electrocardiography

Initially normal, features of right ventricular hypertrophy with right axis deviation and a small P pulmonale become apparent. Bilateral ventricular hypertrophy will develop if ventricular septal defect, patent ductus arteriosus or pulmonary outflow obstruction are present.

2-D echocardiography

The position of the aorta anterior to the pulmonary artery is diagnostic of transposition.

Cardiac catheterization with angiography is the only certain method of defining the possible complex relationships of the various structures. Pressure measurements will demonstrate early increased pressure due to the normal neonatal elevated pulmonary vascular resistance. Persistence of elevated pulmonary vascular resistance, however, suggests the presence of pulmonary outflow tract obstruction. There will be higher oxygen saturation in the pulmonary artery than in the aorta.

The presence of intracardiac shunts, extracardiac shunts or associated cardiac anomalies will also be defined.

Surgical treatment

Palliative

1 *Rashkind procedure (balloon atrial septostomy)*: This procedure is performed upon completion of the initial diagnostic catheterization. The balloon, having been passed through the patent foramen ovale into the left atrium, is inflated and pulled back into the right atrium thereby rupturing the membrane of the foramen ovale and permitting greater intracardiac mixing of blood. This is a life-saving procedure in neonates with an intact ventricular septum.

2 *Blalock–Hanlon procedure*: This is an operative atrial septostomy that is available when balloon septostomy is inadequate, performed through a right thoracotomy.

3 *Banding of pulmonary artery*: The presence of a large ventricular septal defect may cause excessive pulmonary blood flow, which can be reduced by a banding procedure.

4 *Blalock–Taussig shunt*: This procedure may have a place if there is an associated ventricular septal defect and pulmonary stenosis.

Definitive procedures

All procedures are carried out via a midline sternotomy, using extracorporeal circulation with hypothermia and cardioplegia.

Patients with transposition of the great vessels and an intact ventricular septum are candidates for an atrial switch procedure, which is usually done at 4–6 months of age.

Atrial switch procedures

1 *The mustard operation*: A large patch of pericardium is harvested and shaped. The atrial septum is visualized and excised through a right atriotomy.

Commencing to the left of the left pulmonary veins, the tailored patch is sutured into place with 5-0 absorbable sutures. The suture line is carried round the pulmonary veins and the orifices of the venae cavae to the residual septal margin. Inferiorly it is sutured to the eustachian valve. The coronary sinus is left to drain into the new physiological left atrium (Fig. 29.2).

The new left atrium is enlarged with a diamond-shaped patch of pericardium to prevent pulmonary vein obstruction.

Any associated ventricular septal defect is closed transatrially with a patch. If there is pulmonary stenosis, the pulmonary valve is exposed through the pulmonary artery, its leaflets retracted and the subvalvular obstruction excised.

2 *The Senning operation*: The right atrium is incised 5 mm anterior to the sulcus terminalis and extended down to the orifice of the inferior vena cava at the insertion of the eustachian tube. A septal flap is developed; its base extends from the superior aspect of the right superior pulmonary vein to the inferior aspect of the right inferior pulmonary vein for a length of about 3 cm. The flap is lengthened with a patch of pericardium so that it can reach from the left atrial wall to the right atrial wall. The tip of

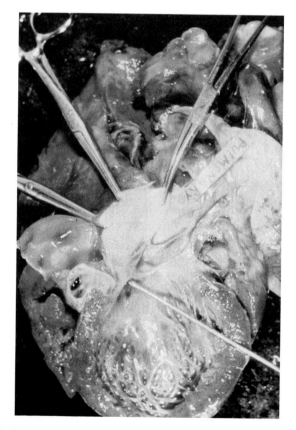

Fig. 29.2. Intracardiac view of transposed aorta and pulmonary artery.

the flap is sutured around the left pulmonary vein orifices with 5-0 synthetic absorbable sutures, after a mattress suture has been placed between the orifices of the left pulmonary veins and the orifice of the left atrial appendage.

The left atrium is now incised longitudinally, as close as possible to the interatrial groove. A lateral incision is made from the midpoint, extending between the right pulmonary veins.

The free edge of the right atrium is sutured to the remnant of the atrial septum and the eustachian valve.

A venting catheter is inserted through the right atrial appendage into the right ventricle.

The anterior edge of the incised right atrium is brought down over the venae cavae and sutured to the posterior edge of the left atrium, using small bites to prevent compression of the venae cavae.

3 *The Rastelli procedure*: Although the atrial switch procedures can be used to manage transposition of the great arteries complicated by ventricular septal defect and left ventricular outflow tract obstruction, the Rastelli procedure is the preferred technique. It converts the left ventricle into the systemic pumping chamber.

The pulmonary artery is transected distal to its valve and the proximal end is oversewn. The right ventricle is incised high along its outflow tract, avoiding injury to the coronary artery.

The ventricular septal defect and the aortic orifice are identified and an intraventricular dacron prosthetic tunnel created between the edge of the septal defect and the aortic orifice, without injuring the conduction pathway.

A conduit of appropriate size is sutured distally to the transected pulmonary artery and, after being trimmed is anastomosed proximally to the edges of the ventriculotomy.

4 *Arterial switch procedure (Jatene procedure)*: This procedure is limited to infants with transposition of the great arteries, a ventricular septal defect and reversible pulmonary hypertension, so that the left ventricle has developed enough contractile force to maintain systemic pressure once the operation is completed.

After exposure of the heart, the aorta is dissected free from the pulmonary artery and its branches. The right and left pulmonary arteries are mobilized to the lung hila and the ligamentum arteriosum is divided.

Cardiopulmonary bypass and deep hypothermia are initiated and the anatomy of the coronary artery origins is defined. The site of their transfer to the pulmonary artery is marked with fine sutures.

The aorta is transected beyond its sinuses, the coronary arteries with a rim of aortic wall are excised and the pulmonary artery is transected.

The pulmonary arteries are incised at the previously marked sites and the cuffed coronary arteries are sutured into place with 6-0 prolene sutures.

The distal pulmonary artery is brought anterior to the aorta. The distal aorta is anastomosed to the proximal pulmonary artery with 5-0 prolene. The distal pulmonary artery is anastomosed to the root of the aorta either directly or by an interposition Gore-tex prosthetic tube graft. Defects created by excision of the coronary ostia are repaired with patches of bovine pericardium.

The Damus–Stansel–Kaye procedure is an arterial switch without coronary artery relocation. The pulmonary artery is transected and the proximal end is anastomosed to the side of the ascending aorta. The aortic valve is closed by suture.

An external conduit is anastomosed proximally to a right ventriculotomy and to the distal pulmonary artery.

Corrected transposition of the great arteries
Embryologic anatomy
Due to an abnormal looping of the primitive embryonic heart tube, the right atrium is connected to the left ventricle from which courses the pulmonary artery. The left atrium connects to the right ventricle and then to the aorta. As a result of the atrioventricular and ventriculo–vascular discordance there has resulted a physiological correction despite the left ventricle pumping to the lungs and the right ventricle to the systemic circulation.

The clinical effects are due to the high incidence of associated intracardiac defects, e.g. ventricular septal defect, pulmonary stenosis or insufficiency of one or other atrioventricular valve:

1   Congestive cardiac failure due to excessive and unrestricted pulmonary blood flow
2   Cyanosis with a systolic murmur due to subvalvular pulmonary stenosis with reduced pulmonary blood flow
3   Syncope due to heart block and rhythm disturbances attributable to the altered course of the conduction system from the A-V node to the ventricular septum.

Radiology

As the aorta is to the left of the pulmonary artery (L-TGA) there is a straight left cardiac border. Cardiomegaly is enhanced by the presence of a VSD.

Electrocardiography

There will be a variable degree of A-V block; WPW syndrome and features of left ventricular hypertrophy.

2-D echocardiography confirms L-TGA and any associated intracardiac anomalies.

Cardiac catheterization and angiography will reveal the architectural arrangement of the heart chambers and great vessels. Ventriculography may be necessary to demonstrate A-V valve incompetence. The left A-V valve may demonstrate Ebstein's anomaly.

Surgical treatment

This is usually determined by the associated intracardiac lesions:

1   *Pulmonary banding* if a large VSD is present without pulmonary stenosis
2   *Blalock shunt* for pulmonary stenosis
3   *Valve reconstruction or replacement* for A-V valve incompetence
4   *Definitive repair:* Closure of VSD and relief of pulmonary outlet obstruction without compromising the integrity of the conduction system. This is best achieved by using an external conduit between the left ventricle and the pulmonary artery without compromising any coronary arteries that run an abnormal course.
5   *Permanent pacemaker for spontaneous heart block*
    a) Transvenous route
    b) Myocardial electrodes at time of VSD closure.

Situs inversus and dextrocardia

Embryology

Rotation of the primitive cardiac loop in the opposite direction to its normal leftward direction will result in dextrocardia with the heart situated in the right chest with the apex pointing to the right and reflecting a "mirror image" of the normal with chamber inversion or corrected transposition of the great vessels.

Dextrocardia

This may exist alone as an isolated dextrocardia, with the heart often suffering associated congenital anomalies such as pulmonary stenosis, persistent truncus arteriosus and transposition of the great arteries, or it may be associated with transposition of the viscera (*situs inversus*).

Situs solitus

This term means that the right–left relationship of the asymmetric viscera and the atria are normal, i.e. the right and left main stem bronchi are normally placed, the right atrium is to the right of the left atrium and the left atrium is to the left. The ventricles are in the normal concordant positions. Ventricular inversion may, however, occur with the right ventricle posterior and to the left of the morphological left ventricle.

Situs inversus

The right to left relationships are the opposite of the normal, i.e. isomerism prevails. Usually the atrial and thoracic viscera are in concordant situs. The right lung has two lobes, the left lung has three lobes. The gall bladder, liver and caecum are on the left and the gastric gas bubble is on the right.

Kartagener's syndrome

In 20% of patients with situs inversus, bronchiectasis and aplasia or inflammation of the frontal sinuses will be present. Congenital cardiovascular anomalies are rarely present.

Situs ambiguus

There is absence of lateralization in the thoracic organs and the atrial chambers. There is usually lack of abdominal lateralization, i.e. asplenia or polysplenia, with the usually asymmetric structures becoming symmetric.

Asplenia

These patients are bilaterally right-sided with right atriopulmonary isomerism, i.e. right-type configuration of main stem bronchus and its pulmonary artery on both sides of the chest.

Polysplenia

These patients are bilaterally left-sided with left atriopulmonary isomerism, i.e. left-type configuration of main stem bronchus and its pulmonary artery bilaterally.

A common atrium is often present in situs ambiguus, with right or left atrial isomerism reflected in the morphology of the atrial appendages. Complex cardiac anomalies may occur in these patients.

Diagnosis of situs inversus

Clinical examination and radiological study will identify the heart to be on the right side. The gastric gas bubble will be seen on the right side while the left dome of the diaphragm will be at a higher level.

Electrocardiography will provide patterns that are a "mirror image" of normal tracings.

Further Reading

Castaneda A. R., Trusler G. A., Paul M. H. *et al.* The early results of treatment of simple transposition in the current era. *J. Thorac. Cardiovasc. Surg.* 95: 14, 1988.

Jatene A. D., Fontes, V. F., Paulista P. P. *et al.* Anatomic correction of transposition of the great vessels. *J. Thorac. Cardiovasc. Surg.* 72: 364, 1976.

Mustard W. T., Keith J. D., Trusler G. A. *et al.* The surgical management of transposition of the great vessels. *J. Thorac. Cardiovasc. Surg.* 48: 953, 1964.

Radley-Smith R., Yacoub M. H. One stage anatomic correction of simple complete transposition of the great arteries in neonates. *Br. Heart J.* 51: 685, 1984.

Rastelli G. C., Wallace R. B., Ongley P. A. Complete repair of transposition of the great arteries with pulmonary stenosis: A review and report of a case corrected by using a new surgical technique. *Circulation* 39: 83, 1969.

Senning A. Surgical correction of transposition of the great vessels. *Surgery* 45: 966, 1959.

Van Praagh R., Van Praagh S., Vlad P., Keith J. D. Anatomic types of congenital dextrocardia: Diagnosis and embryologic implications. *Am. J. Cardiol.* 13: 510, 1964.

Chapter 30
Persistent Truncus Arteriosus

This is a rare congenital anomaly in which septation of the common truncus arteriosus fails to take place, with persistence of a single great vessel which receives blood from both the left and right ventricles. Since the truncal septum plays a role in the normal final closure of the ventricular system, there is always an associated ventricular septal defect.

Anatomical varieties
Type 1
A common trunk arises from the heart. The pulmonary artery comes off the aorta as a result of partial septation and then branches into right and left pulmonary arteries.

Type II
The right and left pulmonary arteries arise separately from the posterior wall of the common aortic trunk.

Type III
The right and left pulmonary arteries arise separately from the lateral walls of the common trunk.

Type IV
No pulmonary arteries arise from the common trunk. Right and left bronchial arteries arise directly from the descending aorta.

Clinical features
1 Central cyanosis is always present, though it may vary in degree. Polycythaemia and clubbing of fingers and toes will develop. Thrombotic phenomena may develop.
2 Congestive cardiac failure: due to diminished pulmonary vascular resistance, heart failure develops within a few weeks after birth. Dyspnoea, tachypnoea, sweating and failure to thrive are associated with cardiomegaly. Pulmonary blood flow is usually increased.

217

3 Systolic ejection murmur: an ejection click may be heard at the
   onset of systole due to the large dilated trunk. The second heart
   sound is unsplit as there is a single set of three or four leaflets
   and not the normal two separate sets of valves.

   The murmur, often associated with a palpable thrill, is best
heard at the 4th interspace to the left of the sternum. A
continuous or diastolic component to the murmur may be
audible due to truncal valve incompetence.

   Radiological examination of the chest demonstrates gross
biventricular cardiomegaly with absence of the pulmonary arc,
leaving a concavity between the enlarged supracardiac aortic
shadow and the left ventricle. The lungs fields are hyperaemic.

   Electrocardiography reflects biventricular hypertrophy and
strain.

   2-D echocardiography delineates a single major vessel arising
from the heart and reveals a ventricular septal defect.

   Cardiac catheterization demonstrates equal pressure in both
ventricles while angiocardiography reveals the specific pattern of
the truncus arteriosus.

Surgical treatment
Operation is postponed as long as possible in patients with mild
symptoms. Most infants have serious symptoms that will lead to
death within 12 months unless successful surgical intervention is
accomplished.

Pulmonary artery banding
As pulmonary hypertension develops early, pulmonary artery
banding was considered to be a valid palliative procedure which
has currently been superseded by immediate primary repair.

Primary repair
Via a midline sternotomy, cardiopulmonary bypass, hypothermia
and cardioplegic arrest are accomplished after occlusion of the
pulmonary artery. The left ventricle is vented.

   The pulmonary trunk is dissected and separated from the aorta
after appropriate clamp control. The aortic opening is sutured.

Alternatively it may be easier to make a vertical aortotomy through which the pulmonary artery ostium is patched and the aortic incision sutured.

The right ventricle is incised just below the truncus and the subaortic ventricular septal defect closed with a dacron patch without injuring the conducting pathway.

A large valved conduit (14–16 mm) is sutured to the pulmonary artery with 5-0 prolene, keeping the valve as close as possible to the pulmonary artery. The proximal prosthesis is then tailored for a 3-0 prolene anastomosis to the ventriculotomy.

Further Reading

Collett R. W., Edwards J. E. Persistent truncus arteriosus: A classification according to anatomic types. *Surg. Clin. N. Am.* 29: 1245, 1949.

Di Donato R. M., Fyfe D. A., Puga F. J. *et al.* Fifteen year experience with surgical repair of truncus arteriosus. *J. Thorac. Cardiovasc. Surg.* 89: 414, 1985.

Ebert P. A., Turley K., Stranger P. *et al.* Surgical treatment of truncus arteriosus in the first 6 months of life. *Ann. Surg.* 200: 451, 1984.

Chapter 31
Total Anomalous Pulmonary Venous Drainage

Embryological anatomy

The pulmonary venous drainage develops at about the third week of gestation. The common pulmonary vein, an outpouching of the common atrium, grows to join the splanchnic plexus which, in turn, communicates with the lung buds, the umbilical, vitelline veins and the cardinal veins.

The venous return to the sinus venosus is transmitted by three paired primitive channels:
1 The vitelline veins which drain the yolk sac
2 The umbilical veins which drain the placenta
3 The cardinal veins which drain the fetus.
The cardinal veins include:
1 Right and left anterior cardinal veins which drain the cephalic region
2 Right and left posterior cardinal veins which drain the trunk and caudal region.

These veins unite to form the common cardinal veins or ducts of Cuvier, which flow into the right and left horns of the sinus venosus.

The right posterior cardinal vein becomes the azygos vein.

A transverse anastomosis between the anterior cardinal veins becomes the left innominate vein.

The left anterior cardinal vein normally obliterates. Failure to obliterate leads to a persistent left superior vena cava.

The right anterior cardinal vein proximal to the left innominate vein becomes the right innominate vein and distally becomes the superior vena cava.

The transverse channel of the sinus venosus persists as the coronary sinus, which provides the venous drainage of the heart.

The right horn of the sinus venosus is absorbed into the right atrium while the left horn remnant persists as the oblique vein of the left atrium.

Pulmonary vein development

The primitive lungs are drained by a venous plexus, which normally loses its connections with the cardinal, umbilical and vitelline veins. The pulmonary venous plexus anastomoses with the two bilateral branches of the common pulmonary vein, which is absorbed into the body of the left atrium. This provides the final normal relationship of four pulmonary veins draining into the left atrium.

Any disruption of these changes will result in the common pulmonary vein draining to the heart via several circuitous pathways, with blood returning from the lungs to the right atrium.

Partial anomalous pulmonary venous drainage

This condition usually affects the right upper pulmonary vein in association with a sinus venosus type of atrial septal defect.

Total anomalous pulmonary connection

Type I: Supracardiac

The common pulmonary vein courses through a vertical venous communication into the left innominate vein and through the superior vena cava to the right atrium.

Type II: Cardiac

The common pulmonary vein drains into the coronary sinus and thus to the right atrium.

Type III: Infracardiac

The common pulmonary vein drains inferiorly through a descending vein that communicates with the portal vein then via the ductus venosus and inferior vena cava to reach the right atrium (Fig. 31.1).

Type IV: Mixed

Components of any of the other three types lead the pulmonary venous drainage directly into the right atrium.

Patent foramen ovale: In total anomalous pulmonary venous drainage some connection between right and left hearts is necessary to sustain life and this is usually mediated by a patent foramen ovale.

Clinical features

Two clinical patterns may manifest.

1 *The restricted pattern*: There is obstruction to the pulmonary venous return to the right atrium, leading to cyanosis which presents early, pulmonary oedema and congestive cardiac failure. The cyanosis is responsive to oxygen administration.

2 *The non-restricted pattern*: The symptoms are delayed, with failure to thrive, growth retardation and recurrent respiratory infections.

   Tachycardia, tachypnoea and hepatomegaly are common. Cyanosis is usually mild in the unrestricted type but is severe and appears early in the neonatal period in the restricted form.

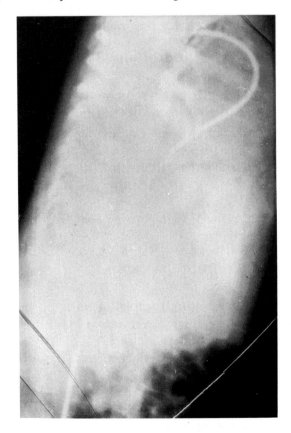

Fig. 31.1. Infracardiac anomalous pulmonary venous drainage defined angiographically.

A soft systolic murmur may be present but is often absent or inaudible.

Without operative intervention, death ensues within 3 months of birth in the restricted group. In the unrestricted group, cardiac failure will cause death within a year in 70% of cases.

Radiological features

Heart size is usually normal. In the supracardiac cases a "figure of eight" or "cottage-loaf" pattern is characteristic.

There is increased pulmonary vascularity due to the increased pulmonary flow. Pulmonary venous congestion is notable in the restricted form due to stenosis of the venous channel.

Electrocardiography

There are features of right ventricular hypertrophy. Right atrial hypertrophy may be reflected in tall peaked P waves in leads II, V1 and V2.

2-D echocardiography may demonstrate the abnormal venous communication.

Cardiac catheterization: a variable degree of pulmonary hypertension will be recorded.

Angiocardiography

Identification of the anomalous venous connection requires the injection of contrast material separately into the right and left pulmonary arteries. Radiographic films will be taken during the venous phase of the pulmonary circulation in order to outline the abnormal venous communication.

Surgical treatment

A midline sternotomy, cardiopulmonary bypass, cardioplegia and deep hypothermia (18–20°C) are utilized in all forms of repair.

Supracardiac type

The apex of the heart is elevated and the ascending common venous channel exposed. After creating a 2 cm incision in the pulmonary venous trunk, the ascending communicating vein is ligated at its origin.

An incision in the left atrium extends from the atrial septum to the base of the left atrial appendage.

The anastomosis is fashioned between the left atrium and the pulmonary venous trunk.

The patent foramen ovale is then closed through a right atriotomy.

Intracardiac type

A right atriotomy permits excision of the intervening septal wall between the atrial septal defect and the coronary sinus, into which the pericardial patch is sutured into place. The atrial septal defect is closed so that the coronary sinus and its pulmonary venous blood empties into the left atrium.

Infracardiac type

In this uncommon type of anomalous pulmonary venous drainage, the descending vein is ligated before it reaches the diaphragm and an anastomosis is created between the left atrium and the common pulmonary venous trunk. A right atriotomy then permits closure of the atrial septal defect.

Scimitar syndrome

The anomalous connection of the right pulmonary vein to the inferior vena cava provides a diagnostic radiological pattern.

A scimitar-shaped vertical shadow, representing the course of the pulmonary vein, is seen alongside the right cardiac border extending to the inferior vena cava.

Patients are usually asymptomatic. Recurrent pulmonary infections and heart failure, due to the left to right shunt, may occur. A soft systolic bruit may be audible.

2-D echocardiography may visualize the vein but venous-phase right pulmonary arteriography may be necessary to confirm the diagnosis.

Surgical treatment

Though infrequently required, it may be necessary in occasional symptomatic cases.

In infants the anomalous vein is detached from the vena cava and is anastomosed to the left atrium.

During extracorporeal circulation a patch is utilized, with creation of a tunnel from the anomalous vein through the atrial septum to the left atrium. The anomalous vein is detached from the inferior vena cava. The caval defect is repaired. A right atriotomy permits a direct anastomosis between the anomalous vein and a small opening created in the right atrial wall.

A small segment of interatrial septum or foramen ovale is excised and a dacron patch fashioned so as to divert the veno-atrial anastomotic flow through the created septal defect into the left atrium.

Cor triatrium

The left atrium is divided into two compartments by a fibrous membrane within which is a small aperture.

Communication between right and left atria is through a patent foramen ovale which may be above or below the membrane.

The left to right shunt that occurs when the foramen ovale is superior to the membrane leads to right ventricular overload, with right heart failure.

If the foramen ovale is inferior to the membrane, pulmonary venous congestion develops.

Children fail to thrive, suffer feeding difficulties and develop congestive heart failure.

Diagnosis

Radiological examination demonstrates prominent pulmonary venous congestion.

Electrocardiography reveals right axis deviation and P wave changes due to right ventricular and right atrial hypertrophy.

2-D echocardiography will visualize the membrane.

Cardiac catheterization demonstrates changes similar to mitral stenosis with pulmonary venous obstruction and pulmonary artery hypertension.

Angiocardiography will outline the two left chambers.

Surgical treatment

Repair is carried out via a midline sternotomy with cardio-pulmonary bypass, hypothermia and cardioplegia.

1   Left atrial approach: this provides good access for excision of the membrane and closure of the foramen ovale.
2   A right transatrial, transseptal approach is preferred in neonates.

Congenital mitral valve stenosis

Isolated congenital mitral stenosis occurs rarely. It may coexist with a patent atrial septal defect (Lutembacher syndrome).

The child will fail to thrive: dyspnoea, tachycardia and an apical diastolic murmur will be noted.

Radiological examination reveals an enlarged left atrium and pulmonary congestion.

2-D echocardiography will confirm the mitral valve stenosis and left atrial enlargement.

Cardiac catheterization will permit assessment of the associated pulmonary hypertension.

Angiocardiography will detail the morphology of the valve, its annulus and the state of the left ventricle. It will also identify associated cardiac defects e.g. Shone's complex (parachute mitral valve, left atrial supravalvular membrane, subaortic stenosis and aortic coarctation).

Surgical treatment

After a period of good medical management with digitalis and diuretics, valve reconstruction or valve replacement may be necessary.

Mitral atresia

2-D echocardiography will reveal a single ventricle below the right atrioventricular valve and absence of the mitral valve.

Survival of the infant depends upon the presence of a large atrial septal defect.

Surgical treatment

Palliative procedures that might be indicated include:
1   Blalock or Glenn shunt if pulmonary blood flow is reduced
2   Pulmonary artery banding if pulmonary blood flow is greatly increased
3   Fontan procedure: the main pulmonary artery is transected and its proximal end closed. An anastomosis is created between the

right atrium and the distal end of the pulmonary artery. The atrial septum is excised and the atrium re-partitioned so that left atrial flow is directed through the single atrioventricular valve into the ventricle.

Further Reading

Edmunds L. H., Wagner H. R. Congenital anomalies of the mitral valve. In: Arciniegas (Ed.), *Paediatric cardiac surgery.* Year Book Medical Publishers. Chicago. 1985.

Hawkins J. A., Clark E. B., Doty D. B. Total anomalous pulmonary venous connection. *Ann. Thorac. Surg.* 36: 548, 1983.

Katz N. M., Kirklin J. W., Pacifico A. D. Concepts and practices in surgery for total anomalous pulmonary venous connection. *Ann. Thorac. Surg.* 25: 479, 1978.

Marks C. *The portal venous system.* Charles C. Thomas Publishers. Springfield. 1973.

Marks C., Albert H. M. Portal-pulmonary venous communication. *J. Cardiovasc. Surg.* 15: 405, 1974.

Murphy J. W., Kerr A. R., Kirklin J. W. Intracardiac repair for anomalous pulmonary venous connection of right lung to inferior vena cava. *Ann. Thorac. Surg.* 11: 38, 1971.

Richardson J. V., Doty D. B., Siewers R. D., Zuberbuhler J. R. Cor triatrium. *J. Thorac. Cardiovasc. Surg.* 81: 232, 1981.

Chapter 32
Congenital Ventricular Disorders

The univentricular heart

Total or partial failure of septation of the primitive ventricle causes clinical features that depend on the amount of pulmonary blood flow.

Excessive pulmonary blood flow

The infant fails to thrive or grow. Minimal cyanosis is associated with congestive cardiac failure. Cardiomegaly and increased pulmonary vascularity are revealed radiologically.

Diminished pulmonary blood flow

Narrowing of the pulmonary outflow tract is associated with a variable degree of cyanosis at birth. Radiologically the heart is small with diminished pulmonary vascularity.

2-D echocardiography: It is important to define whether one or two atrioventricular valves are present and to relate their presence to the semilunar valves. The size of the single ventricular chamber is noted. These facts are important in deciding which operative procedure is preferred.

Cardiac catheterization and angiocardiography should delineate the aortic and pulmonary outflow tracts, with determination of the gradients across the outflow tracts. The exact anatomy of the outflow tracts and their relationships to the large vessels and atrioventricular valves should be delineated angiographically.

Surgical treatment
Septation

The presence of the normal atrioventricular sets of valves is essential for this procedure to be carried out. The septation procedure is especially appropriate in patients with L-transposition of the great vessels. With the aorta to the left, a straight septation patch between the atrioventricular valves corrects the defect.

Although a one-stage septation may be carried out, it may be preferable to accomplish septation in stages, thereby reducing the incidence of conduction block and creating better stability of the neo-septum.

At the first operation the patch is attached loosely with a few sutures to the base and apex of the ventricle, final septation being delayed to a second stage.

Pulmonary artery banding
Though it may relieve pulmonary congestion and cardiac failure, the procedure may complicate subsequent corrective operations.

Modified Norwood procedure
In patients with associated subaortic obstruction, the pulmonary artery is divided and the distal end closed. The proximal end is anastomosed to the aorta, providing a dual aortic flow. A Blalock subclavian–pulmonary conduit restores pulmonary blood flow.

Fontan procedure
An atriopulmonary anastomosis is the procedure of choice in patients with a single atrioventricular valve. The pulmonary valve is occluded by sutures so that all ventricular flow is directed to the aortic opening.

Hypoplastic left heart syndrome
This condition is the most common cause of death due to congenital heart disease in the first month of life.

There is atresia or stenosis of the aortic and mitral valves and hypoplasia of the left ventricle.

Life is sustained by patency of the ductus arteriosus. There is usually an associated coarctation of the aorta.

Clinical features
Blood supply to the body is via the patent ductus arteriosus but circulation to the cerebral and coronary vessels is by retrograde flow, placing such infants in extreme jeopardy.

The child is usually well developed and appears normal at

birth. Within a few hours cyanosis or pallor becomes evident. Inadequate coronary blood flow leads to shock with tachycardia, tachypnoea and signs of cardiac failure. Peripheral pulses are thready and the child has cold clammy extremities.

No murmurs are audible, the first heart sound is normal but there will only be a single second sound, representing closure of the pulmonary valve.

Radiological examination
Cardiomegaly and pulmonary venous congestion are apparent.

Electrocardiography demonstrates right axis deviation in keeping with right ventricular hypertrophy.

2-D echocardiography demonstrates:
1   The hypoplastic left ventricle
2   An hypoplasic ascending aorta and absent aortic valve
3   A small mitral valve.

Treatment
Immediate control of acidosis and renal failure is essential.

Prostaglandin E_1 should be commenced intravenously as soon as the diagnosis is established in order that patency of the ductus arteriosus is maintained.

Surgical management
The Norwood procedure
The operation is carried out via a midline sternotomy using cardiopulmonary bypass, deep hypothermia, cardioplegia and circulatory arrest.

The patent ductus arteriosus is divided. The pulmonary artery is transected and the distal end is oversewn. The hypoplastic aorta is enlarged with a tubular prosthetic patch and the proximal pulmonary artery is incorporated into the aortic anastomosis.

A Blalock subclavian to pulmonary 4 mm Gore-tex shunt is created to provide pulmonary blood flow.

Fontan procedure
At a later reparative stage a right atrial to distal pulmonary artery anastomosis directs blood flow to the lungs. The systemic circulation is sustained by the right ventricle.

Cardiac transplantation
If an appropriate donor becomes available.

Double-outlet right ventricle
The morphological right ventricle gives origin to more than 50% of each great artery. There is an associated perimembranous ventricular septal defect which may be subaortic, subpulmonic or doubly committed in its location. The aorta usually arises to the right and posterior to the pulmonary artery.

If the septal defect is subpulmonic the condition is defined as a Taussig–Bing malformation, with early and severe cyanosis.

If the ventricular septal defect bears no close relationship to either major artery then it is defined as being non-committed.

Radiological examination
Cardiomegaly and marked pulmonary congestion are present.

Electrocardiography
Right or biventricular hypertrophy will be reflected with right axis deviation evident.

2-D echocardiography defines the dual origins of aorta and puimonary artery from the right ventricle and reveals the relationship of the great vessels.

Cardiac catheterization will provide important information regarding pulmonary vascular resistance. Discontinuity between the aortic annulus and the anterior leaflet of the mitral valve is diagnostic.

Angiocardiography defines the dual vascular origins from the right ventricle, identifies the relationship of the arteries to the ventricular septal defect and reveals the architectural arrangement of the double conus with infundibular myocardium beneath the aortic and pulmonary orifices. The aortic and pulmonary valves are seen to be at the same transverse level.

Surgical treatment
Utilizing a midline sternotomy, cardiopulmonary bypass, hypothermia, cardioplegia and a left ventricular vent are established.

The ventricular septal defect may be exposed via a right atriotomy through the tricuspid valve or via a right ventriculotomy.

The size of the VSD should be equal to or larger than the aortic annulus or else it is enlarged anteriorly.

A dacron tube graft is used to create an intraventricular tunnel from the VSD to the aorta using interrupted pledgeted sutures without injuring the conduction system.

If there is an associated pulmonary stenosis, the outflow tract can be enlarged with a patch or a conduit.

In the non-committed VSD where the defect is not closely related to the great vessels, repair may be difficult or impossible.

In the Taussig–Bing malformation with a subpulmonic ventricular septal defect the closure of the VSD creates continuity between the left ventricle and the pulmonary artery, thereby establishing a complete transposition of the great arteries which has to be remedied by one of the following:

1   *Intra-atrial switch:* Mustard or Senning procedure

2   *Rastelli procedure:* Connect VSD to aorta; divide pulmonary artery and conduit from right ventricle to distal pulmonary artery after closure of proximal end.

2   *Arterial switch:* Jatene procedure with coronary translocation or Damus–Stansel–Kaye procedure without coronary translocation.

Further Reading

Anderson R. H., Becker A. E., Tynan M. *et al.* The univentricular atrioventricular connection: Getting to the root of a thorny problem. *Am. J. Cardiol.* 54: 822, 1984.

Bailey L., Concepcion W., Shattuk H., Huang L. Method of heart transplantation for treatment of hypoplastic left heart syndrome. *J. Thorac. Cardiovasc. Surg.* 92: 1, 1986.

Ebert P.A. Staged partitioning of single ventricle. *J. Thorac. Cardiovasc. Surg.* 88: 908, 1984.

Lev M., Bharati S., Meng C. C. L. *et al.* A concept of double outlet right ventricle. *J. Thorac. Cardiovasc. Surg.* 64: 271, 1972.

Norwood W. I., Lang P., Castaneda A. R., Campbell D. N. Experience with operations or hypoplastic left heart syndrome. *J. Thorac. Cardiovasc. Surg.* 82: 511: 1981.

Yacoub M. H., Radley-Smith R. Anatomic correction of the Taussig–Bing anomaly. *J. Thorac. Cardiovasc. Surg.* 88: 380, 1984.

Chapter 33
Anomalous Origin of Left Coronary Artery

The left coronary artery arises abnormally from the posterior aspect of the main pulmonary artery. In time it will steal blood from the right coronary artery as flow proceeds into the lower-pressure pulmonary artery (Fig. 33.1).

At birth the baby appears normal but as the pulmonary artery pressure decreases the child will demonstrate signs of distress, especially during or after feeding:

1   It will clutch at its chest because of angina pectoris.

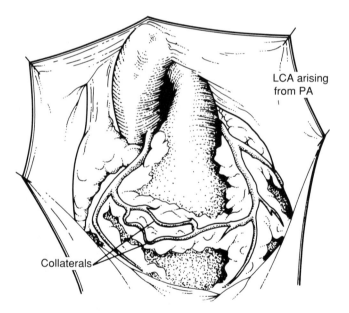

Fig. 33.1. Anomalous origin of left coronary artery from pulmonary trunk.

2 Myocardial infarction: as the pulmonary steal increases, due to inadequate collateral channels, myocardial infarction may develop with subsequent complications e.g. heart failure, ventricular aneurysm or mitral valve insufficiency.

65% of these children will die during the first year of life.

Murmurs are absent unless mitral insufficiency develops.

Radiological examination of the chest may be normal or may reveal post-infarction cardiomegaly.

Electrocardiography will demonstrate ST changes or Q waves with anterolateral myocardial infarction features.

2-D echocardiography demonstrates poor left ventricular contraction.

Aortography will reveal the right coronary artery arising from the aorta, with retrograde filling of the left coronary artery and subsequent opacification of the pulmonary artery.

Cardiac catheterization and left ventriculography may demonstrate a post-infarction aneurysm or mitral valve insufficiency and elevation of left end-diastolic pressure as well as poor left ventricular ejection fraction.

Surgical management
1 Ligation of the left coronary artery at its origin has been done successfully.
2 Revascularization of myocardium using cardiopulmonary bypass:
   a) Reimplantation of left coronary artery into the aorta
   b) Ligation of left coronary artery and aortocoronary bypass graft
   c) Takeuchi operation: an anastomosis between ascending aorta and pulmonary artery with an intrapulmonary graft between the anastomotic orifice and the left coronary ostium
3 Treatment of effects: ventricular aneurysmectomy, repair of destroyed papillary muscle or mitral valve repair.

Coronary artery fistula
There may be an abnormal fistulous vascular channel between a coronary artery and one of the cardiac chambers or the pulmonary artery.

The right coronary artery is most frequently affected, communicating with either the right atrium or the right ventricle.

A continuous precordial murmur is audible in an otherwise asymptomatic child with no specific radiological, electrocardiographic or echocardiographic findings.

Cardiac catheterization and angiography will define the tortuous coronary artery with fistulous communication and opacification of the appropriate cardiac chamber.

Treatment

1 Ligation of the fistulous vessel may be possible without extracorporeal circulation.

2 Under cardiopulmonary bypass the appropriate cardiac chamber is opened and the fistulous orifice closed by suture ligature.

Further Reading

Arciniegas E., Farooki Z. Q., Haimi M., Green E. W. Management of anomalous left coronary artery from the pulmonary artery. *Circulation* 626 (suppl.): 168, 1980.

Crocker D. W., Sobin S., Thomas W. C. Aneurysms of the coronary arteries: Report of three cases in infants and review of the literature. *Am. J. Pathol.* 33: 819, 1957.

Ogden J. A. Congenital anomalies of the coronary arteries. *Am. J. Cardiol.* 22: 474, 1970.

Takeuchi S., Imamura H., Katsumoto K. *et al.* New surgical method for repair of anomalous left coronary artery from pulmonary artery. *J. Thorac. Cardiovasc. Surg.* 78: 7, 1979.

Index

(3)